LLYF
Y COLEG
BAN
NODIANT/NOTATION
RHI
AF606496
COLEG NORMAL BANGOR
3 8052 00060 690 2

Nutritional problems in modern society

Edited by **Alan N. Howard**

John Libbey: London

British Library Cataloguing in Publication Data:

Nutritional problems in modern society
1. Nutrition
612'.3 TX353

ISBN 0-86196-007-6

First published 1981 by

John Libbey & Company Limited
80-84 Bondway, London SW8 1SF

Contents

Preface

This book is addressed to those who have to cope with dietary problems in modern society. The essays deal with *some* of the problems in developed countries. A far wider range of problems of course does exist; indeed it is hoped that if this book is found useful as a companion to the study of human nutrition, a wider selection can be published in a revised edition.

When the Food Education Society held a symposium in London in 1972 entitled 'Nutritional deficiencies in modern society,' it can hardly have been expected that the edited proceedings would still have a readership among students of nutrition seven years later. However this is what happened and the present book is a successor volume.

There are seven entirely new chapters. Chapters which are retained, with some revision, from the earlier work include those on iron deficiency anaemia, vitamin B_{12} and folic acid, vitamin D, and nutritional deficiencies in the elderly.

There are perhaps three main kinds of nutritional problems in 'modern society'. First of all there are the *deficiencies* which occur owing to chance circumstances or poor education. There is the classic problem of *affluence* – obesity – and again the riches and refinements of the modern diet are possibly implicated in the ills which are said to follow from a decline in the consumption of dietary fibre. How many nutritional factors as well as other aspects of health come together is shown in the editor's chapter on coronary heart disease. Lastly there are the problems which particularly must exercise nutritionists and dietitians: *What do we do with the knowledge that we have and how much do we really know?* This comes out strongly in a fascinating chapter about vitamin C by Dr Elwyn Hughes and in the chapters by Dr Darke and Miss Wheeler which deal with dietary assessment and with recommended dietary intakes.

Because this book deals with problems, it does so mainly in a single actual setting, that of the United Kingdom. It is hoped however that readers who are facing nutritional problems in other parts of our 'global village' will still get something of benefit from this book despite its British flavour.

1
Iron-deficiency anaemia

Sheila T. Callender.

Introduction

There is little doubt that iron deficiency is one of the commonest nutritional deficiencies in the world today, affecting large numbers of people in the affluent Western communities as well as those in under-developed countries.

Iron is needed for the manufacture of haemoglobin, the red pigment in the blood which carries oxygen to the organs of the body, and for the muscle pigment myoglobin. It is also contained in the respiratory enzymes of the tissues. Lack of iron leads to anaemia which, if severe, gives rise to symptoms such as tiredness, lack of energy, breathlessness on exertion, and palpitations. A milder degree of anaemia, particularly if it develops slowly, may give rise to little noticeable disturbance because of compensatory processes which lead to more efficient release of oxygen from the haemoglobin.

In addition to the anaemia, various tissue changes may be seen in association with iron deficiency (Chisholm, 1973). The most characteristic change is in the nails which are brittle and in extreme cases become flat and later spoon shaped (Fig. 1). Many patients complain of a sore tongue and there may be obvious atrophy of the papillae leaving the surface of the tongue smooth and redder than normal. Soreness of the corners of the mouth or angular stomatitis may also be seen, particularly in edentulous patients. Difficulty in swallowing referred to the post-cricoid region is another feature associated with iron deficiency and on direct questioning the complaint is elicited in about 20 per cent of patients. In some of these a web of mucosa can be demonstrated on X-ray in the post-cricoid region (the so-called Patterson-Kelly or Plummer-Vinson syndrome). Lack of gastric acid secretion is a further feature in one-third to one-half of the patients with iron deficiency, and changes in the gastric mucosa varying from superficial gastritis to gastric mucosal atrophy are also common.

The epithelial changes are thought, at least in part, to be brought about by deficiency in the iron-containing respiratory enzymes, but associated dietary deficiency or other environmental factors may also play a part. There is no doubt that the epithelial abnormalities were more frequently seen in the 1930s

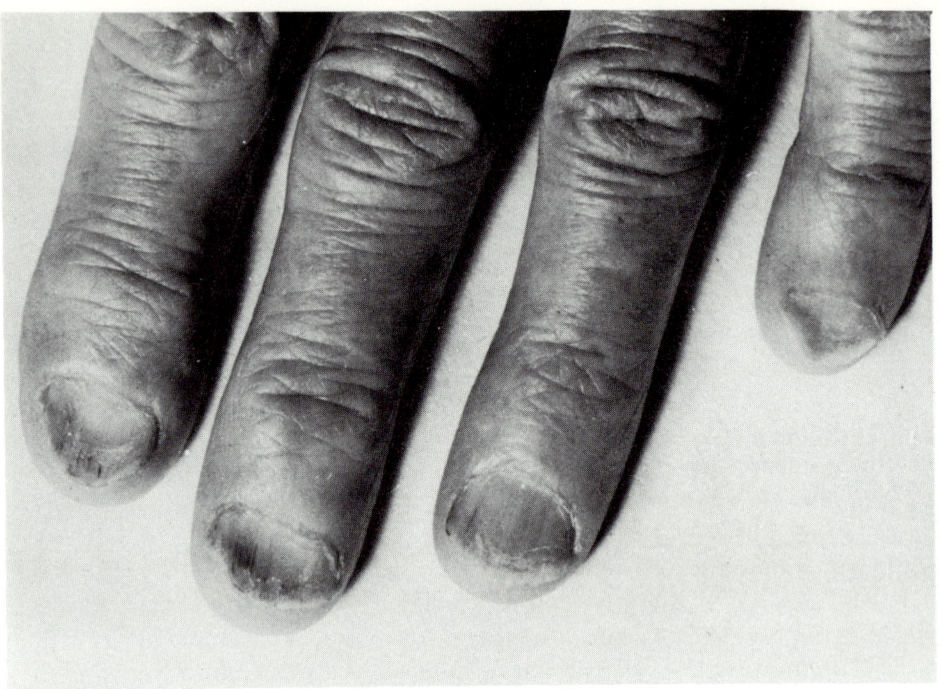

Fig. 1. Koilonychia in long standing iron deficiency

when some of the classical descriptions of iron-deficiency anaemia were made, but there also appears to be good evidence that they have diminished in frequency even during the last 20 years (Chisholm, 1973).

The prevalence of iron deficiency

It is interesting to look back on the papers concerned with the prevalence of iron deficiency in poorer population groups published during the depression of the 1930s. At this time of widespread unemployment, gross poverty, and overcrowding in appalling slums, Davidson and his colleagues found that in Aberdeen 41 per cent of infants, 32 per cent of pre-school children, and 45 per cent of adult women were anaemic. Children of school age and adult males, on the other hand, were seldom anaemic (Davidson *et al.*, 1933; Davidson, Fullerton & Campbell, 1935). About the same time Dr Helen Mackay produced an MRC report on anaemia in infancy in London and this showed a similar very high frequency of iron deficiency in children during the first year of life, and she demonstrated an association between anaemia and increased morbidity (Mackay, 1931).

Many changes have taken place since then. With the last war came full employment and rationing, which did much to improve the average diet in the country as a whole. The National Health Service has made medical care more accessible, and improved standards of living, reduction in the size of families, better ante-natal care and infant welfare services have all played their part in reducing the incidence of iron deficiency.

In spite of all these factors some of the more recent surveys show that iron deficiency is still a common condition in Britain. For example, two studies of random populations in Wales made in 1965 and 1966 showed a prevalence of anaemia in men of 2 per cent and 4 per cent respectively, and in women 12 per cent and 15 per cent (Kilpatrick, 1970). The higher figures in the second survey are thought to reflect the fact that more people over the age of 75 were included and it is beginning to be recognised that this is one of the vulnerable age groups at the present time. A more recent survey (McLennan *et al.*, 1973) among elderly people living at home in the Glasgow area showed that 6 per cent of males and 9 per cent of females over the age of 65 had iron-deficiency anaemia as defined by a haemoglobin of less than 12.0 g/dl and an iron-binding saturation of less than 16 per cent. A further 9 per cent of males and 13 per cent of females had latent iron deficiency with a haemoglobin above 12.0 g/dl but an iron-binding saturation of less than 16 per cent. It is particularly interesting to note that, in this study, poor dietary iron intakes of less than 6 mg/day did not show a correlation with the occurrence of anaemia.

A survey of women in a Glasgow general practice showed an incidence of 9.7 per cent of iron-deficiency anaemia in patients attending the doctor for symptoms, and 2 per cent in subjects seen without complaints. A further 22.2 per cent of 'patients' and 16 per cent of 'subjects' were recognised as having latent iron deficiency; a state where the iron stores are depleted but anaemia has not yet developed (McFarlane *et al.*, 1967).

In other countries in Western Europe surveys have shown a prevalence of between 15 per cent and 25 per cent of iron-deficiency anaemia for women of child-bearing age (Dresch, 1970; Hallberg, 1970; Seibold, 1970; Vellar, 1970).

Iron requirements

Deficiency in iron implies a lack of balance between the intake of iron and the needs of the body.

The body of a 70 kg man contains about 3-4 g of iron, most of which is in the haemoglobin. About 0.5-1g is in storage iron and this can be called upon, for example following haemorrhage, to bring the haemoglobin back to normal. A small but important fraction is in the respiratory enzymes and about 30 mg are in the plasma attached to the iron-binding protein transferrin which carries the iron to and from the various other compartments. Women have rather less iron, both because of their smaller blood volume and lower haemoglobin and because they have less storage iron.

The red cell normally stays in the circulation for about 120 days, after which time it is destroyed. The protein part of the cell is lost from the body but the iron is carefully conserved and goes back to the bone marrow to be used in the manufacture of new red cells. This means that only traces of iron are lost from the body each day in the desquamated cells from the gastrointestinal tract, the skin, and from the urinary tract (Moore, 1964).

This iron loss is regarded as the 'minimal obligatory loss' and it is all that needs to be replaced in the mature man or post-menopausal female. Clearly women during reproductive life have, as a result of the blood loss at menstruation, a greater need for iron, as do pregnant women and growing children.

Infants derive their initial stores of iron from the mother. The bulk of the iron goes to the foetus during the last trimester of pregnancy. Even if the mother herself is short of iron, the iron derived from the breakdown of her cells will go across the placenta to the foetus; this makes her even more anaemic and gives at best an inadequate supply to the child. The baby is born with an excess of red cells and a high haemoglobin, and within the first few weeks of extra uterine life these excess cells are destroyed; the iron thus released goes into stores to help tide the baby over the months of low iron intake from milk.

Babies born prematurely do not have the normal supply of iron at birth and hence become anaemic unless given supplementary iron. Until mixed feeding is established the child has to use up storage iron and if milk feeding goes on too long anaemia is inevitable.

As the child grows the blood volume increases and iron requirements rise. Children, therefore, need to absorb additional iron over and above their minimal daily requirement to remain in balance. A youngster who grows particularly rapidly at any stage may run into deficit although this may only be a temporary state and may adjust itself as growth slows again.

At puberty the iron requirement of girls rises sharply with the onset of menstruation. Swedish workers, as a result of direct measurements of menstrual loss in a random population of women, have shown that the median loss of blood per period is 30 ml. Some women lose far more than this. Those who lose more than 80 ml per period, and this means about 11 per cent of women, have an increased incidence of iron deficiency (Rybo, 1970).

Pregnancy makes additional demands on women for iron, which has to be provided for the foetus, placenta, blood loss at parturition, and also an increase in the red cell mass of the mother which occurs during the last three months of pregnancy. It is true that during pregnancy and lactation iron will not be lost through menstruation, nevertheless the requirement for pregnancy is often in excess of the amount saved.

At the menopause, women's need for iron drops to that of adult men and in this older age group, in the absence of any pathological blood loss, for example from the gastrointestinal tract, the requirement will be no more than that needed to replace the minimal obligatory loss.

In quantitative terms this means that the adult man or post-menopausal woman requires to absorb no more than about 1 mg/day of iron to replace the minimal obligatory loss, but during growth this may be doubled, and in women during reproductive life and notably during the last trimester of pregnancy the requirement may go up to as much as 4 mg/day.

Dietary iron intake

Since even poor diets seldom contain less than 6 mg/day of iron, if all this were available for absorption it would be an easy matter to maintain balance and, indeed, iron overload would be more of a problem than iron deficiency. In fact only a proportion of the iron is absorbed, the amount depending on the interplay of a variety of factors, namely the composition of the diet, the gastrointestinal secretions, the integrity of the gut mucosa, the state of the body iron stores and the rate of erythropoiesis.

Iron in food is present in two principal forms: ferric iron complexes and haem compounds. These two types of iron should be considered separately, both because they are absorbed by a different mechanism, and because they are differently affected by various other factors within the lumen of the gut.

Non-haem iron absorption

The acid which is normally present in the gastric secretion helps to keep ferric iron in solution, and absorption of this type of iron is reduced in subjects with lack of gastric acid. There are also muco-protein substances in the normal gastric secretion which help to form soluble iron chelates, which remain in solution as the food passes on into the alkaline medium of the small intestine (Jacob & Miles, 1969). Substances in the food such as ascorbic acid aid absorption of iron both by their reducing action and by forming soluble low-molecular-weight ligands with iron. Other substances such as phosphates, phytates and tannins reduce absorption by precipitation of the iron.

Haem iron absorption

In the case of haem iron, the haem is split from the protein by digestion and is absorbed into the mucosal cell as haem (Conrad, 1970). Iron is liberated within the mucosal cell and is subsequently passed into the blood stream.

Iron from isolated haem is poorly absorbed; it requires the presence of globin or other protein degradation products and preferably an alkaline medium which prevents the formation of large insoluble polymers. Achloryhdria therefore, if anything, encourages rather than reduces haem iron absorption.

Other factors in the diet such as phytates, phosphates and ascorbic acid do not affect the absorption of haem iron.

Recent recommendations for the daily intake of iron for adults vary from 10-18 mg. It has been pointed out that in general there is a linear relationship between energy and iron in the diet and that the iron content per energy unit of the diet of a population should be adjusted to the requirements of those individuals who have the greatest need for iron, ie the adult female. On this basis Swedish workers feel that diets should be designed to have 10 mg of iron per 1000 kcal (Wretlind, 1970). The daily intake of most people in Western Europe at present is more in the region of 6 mg per 1000 kcal.

This type of figure is, however, not very meaningful for a variety of reasons. First, calculations derived from tables may be grossly misleading because they take no account of the great variation in iron content of foods grown under different conditions, or the iron added in the preparation of foods. The use of iron cooking pots is well known to be associated with an excessively high iron intake in the Bantu of South Africa and this leads to a pathological degree of iron overload (Bothwell, 1964). When iron pots were part of the ordinary kitchen equipment in the United Kingdom they probably also made a significant contribution to the daily iron intake, particularly during the preparation of acid foods.

The contribution of fluids is often not considered in making calculations of dietary intake and many alcoholic drinks, for example, contain significant amounts of iron (MacDonald, 1963; Anguissola, 1970). Even water from deep wells has been found to have up to 5 mg of iron per litre (Moore, 1964).

Iron is more readily absorbed from some foods than others, furthermore foods interact with each other, some aiding iron absorption and others inhibiting. The actual composition of the diet therefore is as important as its total iron content.

Measurements of iron absorption

Chemical iron-balance studies are a logical approach to the investigation of iron retention from whole diets, but they are difficult and time-consuming and require active co-operation from the subjects taking part and meticulous care in the assay of iron in order to avoid contamination.

The introduction of radioactive isotopes of iron concentrated attention on the study of iron absorption from simple iron salts. Although such tests may give valuable information about the maximal capacity of the gut to absorb iron under standard conditions the results do not necessarily reflect the ability to absorb iron from foods.

Much work has been done on evaluation of radio-isotope techniques for biological labelling of foods and for labelling foods *in vitro*. Certain individual foods lend themselves to biological labelling, for example vegetables can be grown in hydroponic tanks with radioactive iron added to the nutrient media, and animals may be injected with radioactive iron which they will build into their tissues and blood or, in the case of birds, incorporate into their eggs.

Studies of iron absorption from foods which have been labelled biologically have shown great variability in absorption (Layrisse, Martinez-Torres & Roche, 1968; Layrisse *et al.*, 1969; Callender, 1971). Iron in meat, fish and haemoglobin is well absorbed, that from vegetables and cereals much less well, the exception being iron in soya beans which is comparatively well absorbed (Fig. 2). Iron in eggs is present as a phosphoprotein complex from which it is very poorly absorbed (Callender, Marney & Warner, 1970).

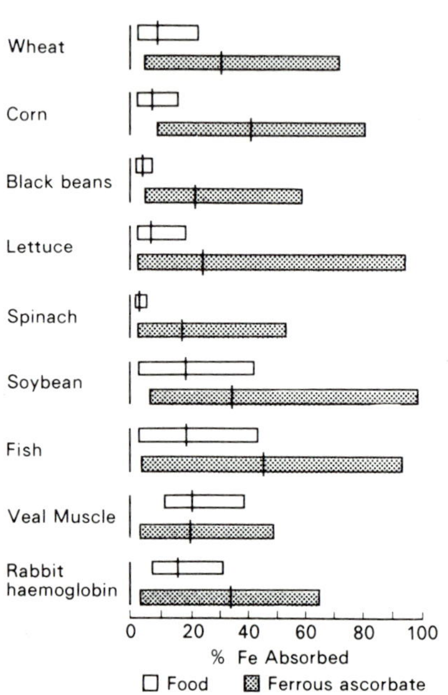

Fig. 2. Iron absorption from foods labelled biologically with radioactive iron compared with absorption from ferrous ascorbate in the same subjects. A double isotope technique was used measuring the comparative absorption (Data from Layrisse *et al.*, 1969)

Clearly, biological labelling with radioactive iron has limitations, hence the interest in validating the results of tests of iron absorption from foods which have been labelled *in vitro* (Bjorn-Rasmussen *et al.*, 1974).

Some foods can have the radio-isotope incorporated during preparation before cooking, for example radioactive iron can be added to flour before baking into bread or cakes. This is particularly useful in investigating the efficacy of fortification of foods with iron.

The majority of studies have, however, been made by mixing the tracer radioactive iron with an individual food or a meal after cooking. When a tracer dose of iron labelled with either ^{59}Fe or ^{55}Fe is mixed with a food labelled biologically with the alternative isotope of iron the ratio between the absorption from the two isotopes has been found to be close to unity over a wide range of absorption, suggesting that the 'external tag' enters into a non-haem iron pool and reflects accurately the iron absorption from this compartment.

Similar studies using haem iron as the 'external tag' and meat labelled biologically with radioactive iron as the 'internal tag' have suggested that the 'external tag' of haemoglobin iron mixes fully with the haem pool. Using two external tags it is possible therefore to measure the net absorption of haem and non-haem iron from a complete meal.

It appears that if the radioactive tracer is added either drop by drop to the prepared meal or is mixed in with the main bulky component a satisfactory estimate of the iron absorption from the haem or non-haem iron in the meal (depending on the tag used) is obtained. If the radioactive tracer is simply taken as a drink through the meal absorption may be over-estimated.

Iron absorption from foods may be favourably or unfavourably influenced by other foods (Fig. 3), for example 100 ml of orange juice or 100 grams of raw

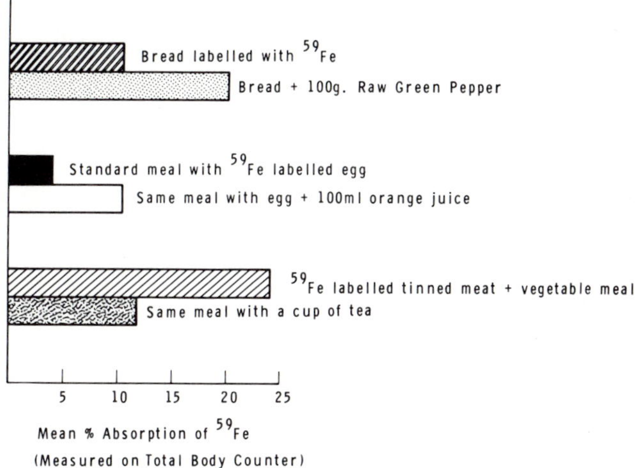

Fig. 3. The effect of interaction of foods on iron absorption

green pepper is sufficient to enhance absorption of non-haem iron from such foods as eggs and bread, presumably because of their high ascorbic-acid content. Conversely eggs reduce iron absorption from other non-haem iron in foods and perhaps most significantly the drinking of tea with a meal reduces iron absorption (Disler *et al.*, 1975).

Animal protein, as for example in meat, will enhance iron absorption from vegetable sources as well as increasing the absorption of iron from haemoglobin.

From these examples it is evident that it is difficult to predict exactly what proportion of the daily dietary iron an individual will absorb. From the earlier chemical iron balance studies on a mixed type of diet 10-14 per cent of the iron appeared to be absorbed. This, on a diet containing 10-15 mg of iron, would just cover the minimal obligatory loss of the adult male and post-menopausal female, but studies of the absorption from individual foods have shown that in non-anaemic individuals the iron absorption is usually considerably less than 10 per cent.

One of the most interesting facets of iron absorption concerns the way in which the body can adjust the amount of iron absorbed according to its needs and, indeed, a test of iron absorption is regarded as being one of the most sensitive indices of the state of the body iron stores. Absorption of simple ferrous iron salts can be increased up to four-fold but iron absorption from foods is not, as a rule, more than doubled or trebled (see Table 1). Such an adjustment may be sufficient to restore the iron balance provided the iron losses are not excessive and the diet contains a good proportion of meat and haemoglobin. There are, however, limits to this adjustment and it is unlikely that the 11 per cent of women who have excessive menstrual loss could ever meet their requirements from the diet alone.

Table 1. Iron absorption in normal and iron deficient subjects

		Mean % of iron absorbed	
		Normal	**Iron deficiency**
Ferrous ascorbate (5mg Fe)		9.2	40.1
*White bread	Included in	2.2	7.3
Oat cakes and porridge	a standard	4.0	10.0
Eggs	meal plus tea	2.2	5.6
Chicken muscle		6.9	17.0
Haemoglobin		10.0	22.0

*Labelled with ^{59}Fe *in vitro*

Fortification of food with iron

There is much current interest in proposals for tackling the problem of widespread iron deficiency by fortification of food. This is certainly effective in certain circumstances, for example the development of iron deficiency in premature infants can be prevented by the fortification of the milk formula with iron to about 12 mg per quart (Gorten, 1965). Several countries already have a policy of adding iron to flour, and at present in the United Kingdom flour of less than 80 per cent extraction has iron added to bring the level to 1.65 mg per 100 grams of flour. From studies of iron absorption from bread calculations as to the possible contribution to the positive iron balance from this source indicate that this is not a very profitable approach (see Table 2) (Callender & Warner, 1971). The studies on which these calculations were based were made

Table 2. Estimated contribution of bread to the daily iron balance in the UK (Ministry of Agriculture, Fisheries and Food, 1965)

Daily iron intake from bread*	1.8 –2.6mg
Absorption from added iron	0.01 – 0.02mg
Absorption from natural iron	0.07 – 0.10mg
Absorption from whole meal bread	0.10 – 0.15mg

on subjects who substituted bread labelled with ^{59}Fe for normal bread and used it as part of their ordinary diet. No attempt was made to control the intake of other constituents of the diet. The natural iron in wholemeal flour may be somewhat better absorbed than that added to white flour, and a return to lower extraction flour may be desirable.

In some countries with programmes for widespread fortification of food with iron, concern is being expressed about the potential hazard of iron overload. In this country probably little harm would accrue from increasing the iron intake within limits. The dietary iron overload which occurs in the Bantu in South Africa is the result of an unusually high daily intake of 100-200 mg of iron, associated with the consumption of Kaffir beer. Alcohol may increase the absorption of iron and cirrhosis of the liver, which may result from chronic alcoholism, may also be associated with increased iron absorption. In countries with a high intake of alcohol, therefore, high dietary iron is potentially hazardous.

In other countries such as those of south-east Asia, and Cyprus, there is a high incidence of thalassaemia, a condition in which the absorption of iron tends to be inappropriately high and iron overload may cause premature death. Although numerically the incidence of iron loading disease is much less than that of iron deficiency, iron overload is potentially lethal whereas iron deficiency gives rise to morbidity rather than mortality. Hence any benefit of iron fortification programmes should be weighed up carefully against possible harm which they might cause.

Conclusion

In conclusion, there is no doubt that iron deficiency is a widespread problem, but in this country the incidence has been reduced by better medical care and better standards of living. It is difficult to change people's dietary traditions, but attempts should be made to educate the public about the foods which are beneficial from the point of view of iron nutrition, notably meat and haemoglobin products, the usefulness of citrus fruits in aiding absorption, and the avoidance of drinking tea with meals.

Fortification of food with iron probably has a limited application, but the alternative approach of detection of iron deficiency and treatment of those at risk, as is already widely done during pregnancy and in infancy, would seem to be safer and more profitable.

**Later figures (1976) show the same mean daily contribution of iron from bread, ie 2.2 mg*

References

Anguissola, A.B. (1970): Nutritional value of wine. In *Iron deficiency,* ed L. Hallberg, H.-G. Harwerth and A. Vannotti, p.71. London and New York: Academic Press.

Bjorn-Rasmussen, E., Hallberg, L., Isaksson, B. & Arvidsson, B. (1974): *J. Clin. Invest.* 53, 247.

Bothwell, T.H. (1964): Iron overload in the Bantu. In *Iron metabolism,* ed F. Gross, p. 362. Berlin: Springer.

Callender, S.T. (1971): *Geront. Clin.* 13, 44.

Callender, S.T., Marney, S.R. & Warner, G.T. (1970): *Br. J. Haemat.* 19, 657.

Callender, S.T. & Warner, G.T. (1971): *Haematologica* 5, 369.

Chisholm, M. (1973): Tissue changes associated with iron deficiency. In *Clinics in haematology* 2, p. 203. London: Saunders.

Conrad, M. (1970): Factors affecting iron absorption. In *Iron deficiency*, ed. L. Hallberg, H.-G. Harwerth and A. Vanotti, p. 87. London and New York: Academic Press.

Davidson, L.S.P., Fullerton, H.W., Howie, J.W., Croll, J.M., Orr, J.B. & Godden, W. (1933): *Br. Med. J.* 1, 685.

Davidson, L.S.P., Fullerton, H.W. & Campbell, R.M. (1935): *Br. Med. J.* 2, 195.

Disler, P.B., Lynch, S.R., Charlton, R.W., Torrance, J.D., Bothwell, T.H., Walker, R.B. & Mayet, F. (1975): *Gut* 16, 193.

Dresch, C. (1970): Prevalence of iron deficiency in France. In *Iron deficiency* ed L. Hallberg, H.-G. Harwerth and A. Vannotti, p. 423. London and New York: Academic Press.

Gorten, M.K. (1965): *Am.J. Clin. Nutr.* 17, 322.

Hallberg, L. (1970): Prevalence of iron deficiency in Sweden. In *Iron deficiency,* ed L. Hallberg, H.-G. Harwerth and A. Vannotti, p. 453. London and New York: Academic Press.

Jacobs, A. & Miles, P.M. (1969): *Br. Med. J.* 4, 778.

Kilpatrick, G.S. (1970): Prevalence of iron deficiency in the United Kingdom, In *Iron deficiency,* ed L. Hallberg, H.-G. Harwerth and A. Vannotti, p. 441. London and New York: Academic Press.

Layrisse, M., Martinez-Torres, C. & Roche, M. (1968): *Am.J.Clin. Nutr.* 21, 1175.

Layrisse, M., Cook, J.D., Martinez, C., Roche, M., Kuhn, I.N., Walker, R.B. & Finch, C.A. (1969): *Blood* 33, 430.

MacDonald, R.A. (1963): *Arch Intern. Med.* 112, 184.

McFarlane, D.B., Pinkerton, P.H., Dagg, J.H. & Goldberg, A. (1967): *Br. J. Haemat.* 13, 790.

Mackay, H.M.M. (1931): *Nutritional anaemia in infancy with special reference to iron deficiency.* Med. Res. Counc. Spec. Rep. Ser. No. 157. London: HMSO.

McLennan, W.J., Andrews, G.R., Macleod, C. & Caird, F.I. (1973): *Q. Jl Med.* 42, 1.

Moore, C.V. (1964): Iron nutrition. In *Iron metabolism,* ed F. Gross, p. 241. Berlin: Springer.

Rybo, G. (1970): Menstrual loss of iron. In *Iron deficiency,* ed L. Hallberg, H.-G. Harwerth and A. Vannotti, p. 163. London and New York: Academic Press.

Seibold, M. (1970): Prevalence of iron deficiency in Germany. In *Iron deficiency,* ed L. Hallberg, H.-G. Harwerth and A. Vannotti, p. 427. London and New York: Academic Press.

Vellar, O.D. (1970): Prevalence of iron deficiency in Norway. In *Iron deficiency*, ed L. Hallberg, H.-G. Herwerth and A. Vannotti, p. 447. London and New York: Academic Press.

Wretlind, A. (1970): Food iron supply. In *Iron deficiency,* ed L. Hallberg, H.-G. Harwerth and A. Vannotti. London and New York. Academic Press.

2

Dietary deficiency of vitamin B_{12} and folic acid

I. Chanarin.

Vitamin B_{12}

Introduction

Vitamin B_{12} is absent from all foods of plant and vegetable origin. Periodic reports of the assay of small amounts of vitamin B_{12} in alfalfa, pulses, turnip greens, comfrey etc. are explainable in terms of soil contamination. The activity of soil bacteria leads to the presence of small but significant amounts of vitamin B_{12} in soil and natural water supplies. Apart from soil contamination, bacterial fermentation as in stored ground nuts has resulted in a rising vitamin B_{12} content although the freshly harvested nuts are devoid of vitamin B_{12} (Ford & Holdsworth, 1965). The nitrogen-fixing bacteria in the nodules on the roots of legumes contain vitamin B_{12}, but this is not present in the plant itself. Thus, there is no vitamin B_{12} in cereals and hence none in flour, rice and bread; nor in otherwise nutritious foods such as nuts and potatoes. On the other hand vitamin B_{12} is present in some higher plants such as algae, in bacteria and in all foods of animal origin.

Human milk contains 0.4 μg of vitamin B_{12} per litre and cow's milk 3.2 μg per litre.

The total amount of vitamin B_{12} supplied daily in a mixed diet is shown in Table 1. A mixed diet supplying an adequate amount of proteins and energy is likely to contain 4 μg or more of vitamin B_{12}. There is, however, much less information about the vitamin B_{12} content of vegetarian diets. The 'vegetable' components themselves do not supply any vitamin B_{12}. Water used in preparing the food may supply trace amounts. Pre-prepared food may acquire a bacterial flora which may add further vitamin B_{12}. Many vegetarians do take milk or yogurt and some take eggs. Such diets are likely to contain reduced but adequate amounts of vitamin B_{12}. Stewart, Roberts & Hoffbrand (1970) collected a week's prepared diet taken by an Indian lactovegetarian and found a total vitamin B_{12} content of 3.5 μg (0.5 μg per day). Another patient studied by the author had a daily intake of 1.3 and 1.6 μg vitamin B_{12} over two 24-hour periods.

Table 1. Estimates for daily vitamin B_{12} intake

Author	Qualification	Vitamin B_{12} μg/day	
Estren *et al.*, 1958	–	5	
Jolliffe & Peterman, 1956	–	6	
Grasbeck, 1960	–	7	
Chung *et al.*, 1961	3013 kcal & 130g protein	31.6	(4.1 – 85.5)
" "	2439 kcal & 116g protein	16.0	(1.2 – 75.6)
" "	1117 kcal & 31g protein	2.7	(1.1 – 8.1)
Feeley & Moyer, 1961*	48 – 88g protein	3.9 – 4.5	
" "	18 – 22g protein	0.7 – 1.1	
Lowenstein *et al.*, 1966	73g protein	5.7 – 6.4	
Jagerstad *et al.*, 1975 *a*	men 70g protein	5.2	
	women 53g protein	5.6	

*Dietary intake of pre-adolescents

Availability of dietary vitamin B_{12}

The availability of dietary vitamin B_{12} for absorption in man was tested by Heyssel *et al.* (1966). By feeding ^{60}Co as the sole source of cobalt to sheep they induced the synthesis of labelled vitamin B_{12} in the rumen and hence the absorption and deposition in the tissues of the sheep of labelled vitamin B_{12}. Liver and muscle of the animal was then given to volunteers to test the absorption of the vitamin. These studies showed that the vitamin was absorbed to the same extent as a similar dose in aqueous solution. Vitamin B_{12} in food is stable and not affected by heat nor by variation in pH other than extreme alkalinity.

There is however a physiological limitation to the amount of vitamin B_{12} that can be taken up by man from a single oral dose. A maximum of 2-3 μg is taken up from a single meal and this applies equally to vitamin B_{12} in solution as well as the natural vitamin B_{12} in foodstuffs (Swendseid, Gasster & Halsted, 1954). The explanation for the limitation of vitamin B_{12} uptake is uncertain but is probably related to saturation of available receptor sites in the ileum for the vitamin B_{12} intrinsic factor complex. Thus 2-3 μg vitamin B_{12} can be absorbed from a single meal and possibly three times this amount, up to 9 μg, from three meals throughout the day.

Vitamin B_{12} requirement

To maintain the *status quo*, requirement should equal the amount of vitamin B_{12} lost and degraded in the body each day. Observations on vitamin B_{12} loss have been obtained by giving radioactive vitamin B_{12} to man and following its loss from the body generally by whole body counting. Following a period during which it is assumed that the tracer dose equilibrates with the total vitamin B_{12} store, there is a steady loss of the label from the body and this has been accepted as an index of daily vitamin B_{12} loss. This loss is set out in Table 2 and is of the order of 2 to 4 μg daily.

The time lag before the development of vitamin B_{12} deficiency following total gastrectomy has been used as a means of calculating vitamin B_{12} losses. Difficulties in this approach are that there may be a very long lag between the appearance of blood changes and decline of vitamin B_{12} stores. Rate of loss of vitamin B_{12} may vary and be smaller as vitamin B_{12} stores decline. Nevertheless such calculations support a daily loss of between 1.6 to 6 μg daily (Gräsbeck, 1960).

Table 2. Daily loss of vitamin B_{12} in man

	μg*
Grasbeck *et al.*, 1958	1.6 – 6
Bozian *et al.*, 1963	4.8
Heinrich, 1964	2.55
Glass & Lee, 1966	4 – 6.5
Reizenstein *et al.*, 1966	1.2 – 2.0
Adams & Boddy, 1968	2.4 – 7.8

*Based on total vitamin B_{12} stores of 3 – 5 mg

Another parameter that has been looked at in relation to vitamin B_{12} requirement is the amount needed to produce a haematological response. Serial studies by Adams *et al.* (1968) showed that a daily parenteral dose in excess of 1 μg vitamin B_{12} is required to elicit an optimal response in untreated megaloblastic anaemia due to vitamin B_{12} deficiency. Nevertheless, suboptimal responses may be obtained with much smaller amounts; nor is there any means of equating these amounts with the normal daily requirement.

A group set up by the World Health Organisation and the Food and Agriculture Organisation of the United Nations recommend a daily vitamin B_{12} intake of 0.3 μg in the first year of life, 0.9 μg at 1 to 3 years, 1.5 μg at 4 to 9 years, 2.0 μg over the age of 10, 3.0 μg during pregnancy and 2.5 μg during lactation (FAO/WHO report, 1970)

Nutritional vitamin B_{12} deficiency

An inadequate dietary intake of vitamin B_{12} is only possible in subjects taking a fairly strictly vegetarian diet, that is, taking no eggs and very little or no milk. In the UK such subjects are dietary faddists (vegans) or are Indians who for religious reasons are life-long vegetarians.

In a survey of 26 vegans, Ellis & Montegriffo (1970) found a lower mean serum vitamin B_{12} than in controls (236 v 441 pg/ml) but a higher serum folate in the vegans (14.1 vs 5.2 ng/ml). There was no difference in the clinical states of the two groups. Nevertheless vitamin B_{12} neuropathy has been reported by Badenoch (1954) and Smith (1962).

In recent years there has been large scale immigration into the UK of subjects of Indian origin from East Africa. Many of these are strict vegetarians and this group is of particular interest because tropical sprue, which is frequent in India, is uncommon in East Africa. The very difficult differential diagnosis in patients coming from India may be between nutritional vitamin B_{12} deficiency alone or accompanied by tropical sprue. Stewart *et al.* (1970) reported 13 patients with megaloblastic anaemia due to nutritional vitamin B_{12} deficiency. Twelve were Hindu vegetarians. In one patient studied in detail there was a good haematological response to oral treatment with 1μg vitamin B_{12} daily proving that the deficiency was due to failure of dietary intake of vitamin B_{12}.

The frequency of megaloblastic anaemia among Indian immigrants to Britain has been found to be about three times that in white persons (Britt, Harper & Spray, 1971). The commonest cause of the megaloblastic anaemia is nutritional deficiency and in four out of 25 cases this was attributed to vitamin B_{12} deficiency and in a further seven to a mixed deficiency of folate and vitamin B_{12}.

Long-standing vegetarianism as seen in many Hindus leads to low serum vitamin B_{12} levels which may be below 100 pg/ml in half the subjects. The great majority of these subjects are perfectly fit and of similar height and weight to control groups taking a mixed diet (Mehta, Rege & Satoskar, 1964). Thus the finding of a low serum vitamin B_{12} level as the sole abnormal finding in a vegetarian, although an index of reduced vitamin B_{12} stores, is not of clinical significance. Nor are such patients at particular risk in pregnancy, since this makes very little impact on vitamin B_{12} status of the mother (Chanarin, 1969).

Folate

Dietary intake

Some of the earlier observations on folate content of foodstuffs were carried out before the importance of protecting unstable compounds was appreciated. This applies to the data reported by the US Department of Agriculture (Toepfer *et al.*, 1951; Thenen, 1975). Forty diets collected by ten Canadian women had a mean total folate content of 242 μg per day with a range of 60 to 601 μg Moscovitch & Cooper, 1973). A Swedish study gave a daily folate intake of 160 μg/day for women and 410 μg/day for men (range 30 to 1536 μg) (Jagerstad, Lindstrand & Westesson, 1975), and a UK study 129 to 300 μg daily (Chanarin, 1974).

The folate analogues present in a mixed diet are largely methylated derivatives of reduced forms of folic acid, that is, tetrahydrofolic acid and dihydrofolic acid and the bulk of these have a long glutamic acid chain, that is, they are polyglutamates. Such analogues comprise more than 50 per cent of dietary folate (Perry, 1971). The second major group were formyl derivatives of reduced forms of folate once again mainly polyglutamates and these comprised 30 per cent of dietary folate.

The predominance of reduced folate derivatives renders dietary folate sensitive to oxidation and the predominance of methyl forms explains the much higher assay values obtained with *L. casei* assay. Cooking too has an adverse effect on folate as does sunlight. The values for dietary folate quoted were obtained on diets after cooking.

Availability of dietary folate

Some 80 per cent of an oral dose of tritium labelled pteroylglutamic acid is absorbed by man (Anderson *et al.*, 1960). Other more physiological analogues are absorbed more completely, less than 5 per cent of labelled material being recovered from the faeces.

There is considerably more uncertainty about the extent to which polyglutamates are absorbed. Studies with ^{14}C-labelled synthetic pteroylpolyglutamate have found about 60–70 per cent absorption of this compound (Butterworth, Baugh & Krumdieck, 1969; Rosenberg & Godwin, 1971). However natural polyglutamate (usually yeast extract) have not produced as satisfactory haematological responses as equimolar amounts of monoglutamate (Perry & Chanarin, 1968). The explanation for this discrepancy is not clear. Natural inhibitors to the enzyme responsible for splitting the glutamic chain from polyglutamate during intestinal absorption have been suggested as an explanation but even the existence of such enzyme inhibitors are in doubt (Hoffbrand, 1969). Should 70 per cent of the polyglutamate in a mixed diet be absorbed this would imply that if a diet contains 300 μg folate, of which 200 is polyglutamate, some 140 μg is absorbed as well as 95 per cent or 95 μg of the monoglutamate. Thus total absorption from such a diet is 235 μg.

Folate requirement

A relatively folate-free diet taken by a well-nourished volunteer led to the appearance of early megaloblastic changes in the marrow after 133 days (Herbert, 1962*a*). On the basis of a total folate body content of 20 mg this indicates a daily folate loss of 150 μg/day. However, the loss of folate occurs at a much more rapid rate in the earlier phases of deprivation and is much slower subsequently (Chanarin, Smith & Winocour, 1969). Thus, turnover of folate may be much greater in the earlier phases of such a study, perhaps 200 to 300 μg daily, and much smaller later on. The validity of such studies as an indication of folate stores and indirectly, requirement, is supported by similar studies in alcoholic subjects who have reduced folate stores. In these megaloblastic changes following presumed depletion of folate stores developed much sooner than in Herbert's study (Eichner, Pierce & Hillman, 1971).

Similarly, the dose of folate required to produce a haematological response in patients with normal folate requirement and with a folate deficient megaloblastic anaemia is 200 μg daily (Hansen & Weinfeld, 1962). An oral dose of 100 μg folate daily was insufficient to prevent a fall in the serum folate values of subjects on very low folate intakes (Herbert, 1962*b*). Thus these data suggest that a daily folate requirement in excess of 100 μg daily and perhaps 200 μg may be a reasonable minimum value. These figures are higher than often quoted, but a FAO/WHO working party (1970) suggested the following values: 0–6 months of age, 40 μg folate daily; 7–12 months, 60 μg; 1–12 years, 100 μg; 13 years and over, 200 μg; pregnancy, 400 μg; lactation, 300 μg.

Two studies have shown that in pregnancy a daily supplement of 100 μg pteroylglutamic acid daily in subjects on a mixed diet is required to maintain the red cell folate level throughout pregnancy (Hansen & Rybo, 1967; Chanarin *et al.*, 1968). When 50 μg was given daily, the red cell folate level continued to decline, whereas with 200 μg daily there was a continued rise throughout pregnancy. Thus on this basis the normal requirement of 200 μg daily increases to 300 μg in pregnancy.

Nutritional folate deficiency

In the UK nutritional folate deficiency may be met with in three population groups: (a) premature infants, (b) pregnant women, (c) the elderly.

Megaloblastic anaemia is not uncommon in premature infants (Zuelzer & Ogden, 1946; Gray & Butler, 1965). Strelling *et al.* (1966) reported a frequency of seven out of 54 babies and suspected it in a further four, and Vanier & Tyas (1967) found anaemia in three out of 20 premature infants who responded to folic acid therapy.

Matoth *et al.* (1964) first pointed out that the whole blood folate levels of breast-fed infants were substantially higher than that found in bottle-fed infants.

At birth, both red cell and serum folate levels are relatively high. These fall steadily to reach the lowest levels at 6–8 weeks. This fall is due to the transition from an abundant folate environment *in utero* to poor folate environment in post-natal life (Shojania & Gross, 1964; Roberts *et al.*, 1969). The lowest serum folate levels were encountered in the smallest infants, particularly the prematures weighing less than 1.7 kg. The explanation for the greater liability of premature infants to megaloblastic anaemia is multifactorial. Folate stores accumulated *in utero* are less than in full-term infants, as judged by lower folate blood levels. Rapid growth is associated with increased folate requirement; but, from the practical viewpoint, their dietary intake appears less adequate than that obtained by a breast-fed infant and less than that required to meet their needs.

Milk, human or bovine, contains 50 μg folate per litre (Ghitis, 1966; Karlin *et al.*, 1967). Heating of the milk results in 40 per cent loss of folate and re-heating or heating of pasteurised milk destroys 80 per cent of the folate content. A not uncommon procedure in paediatric practice was (and perhaps still is) to make up all milk feeds in the morning with heat and to re-heat when the milk is to be given. Many powdered milks on the market may too have very low folate content. Thus an inadequate dietary intake of folate is the important precipitating cause of megaloblastic anaemia in prematurity.

The frequency of megaloblastic anaemia in pregnancy is perhaps the most sensitive index of the nutritional folate status of a population. The additional amount of folic acid required to meet the requirements of a single pregnancy probably does not vary a great deal from person to person. How this stress is met, however, is determined by the folate status before pregnancy and by the folate intake during pregnancy.

Those women who show a megaloblastic anaemia or megaloblastic haemopoiesis in late pregnancy have evidence of nutritional folate deficiency in the early stages of pregnancy and this is the result of nutritional folate deficiency before entering pregnancy. Thus both red cell folate and serum folate levels are significantly lower in early pregnancy in those women who become megaloblastic than in controls who remain normoblastic throughout pregnancy (Chanarin *et al.*, 1968); Temperley, Meehan & Gatenby, 1968). The mean serum folate at the first visit to the ante-natal clinic was 2.0 ng/ml in those who became megaloblastic as compared to a mean of 5.4 ng/ml in controls. Women showing a fall in red cell folate throughout pregnancy had a mean dietary folate intake of 479 μg per 24 hours on direct assay, as compared to another group whose red cell folate levels rose during pregnancy and who had a dietary folate intake of 1019 μg folate per 24 hours (Chanarin, 1969).

The frequency of megaloblastic anaemia, and hence of significant folic acid deficiency, in pregnancy in the UK varied from five in 1000 pregnancies in Scotland, 28 per 1000 in the Midlands, to 54 per 1000 among the Irish in Liverpool. Those figures will have been reduced considerably by widespread use of oral folate supplements in pregnancy, but nevertheless they remain valid as indicating a small but significant degree of folate deficiency in the population. A more sensitive index is the appearance of megaloblastic haemopoiesis on marrow examination and this appears in the surprisingly high number of 25 per cent of pregnant healthy women (Chanarin, 1969).

An interesting seasonal incidence for megaloblastic anaemia in Dublin was noted by Gatenby (1956) and confirmed by others in the UK. Thus, in London, Chanarin (1969) carried out some 200 marrow biopsies over a 2-year period. Fifteen per cent of marrows were megaloblastic during January to March as compared to 5 per cent in October to December. The higher frequency of megaloblastic haemopoiesis in those women who were pregnant during the winter months is almost certainly the result of a much poorer availability of vegetable sources of folate at that time.

Table 3. Folate deficiency in the elderly (UK)

	Low serum folate %	Normal range above x ng/ml	Low RBC folate %	Normal range above x ng/ml
Read *et al.*, 1965	80	5.9	–	–
Hurdle & Williams, 1966	39	5	–	–
Varadi & Elwis, 1966	17	3	14	160
Batata *et al.*, 1967	20	2.1	–	–
Girdwood *et al.*, 1967				
Controls	8	3	–	–
Geriatric	18	–	–	–
Elwood *et al.*, 1971	3	3	8.1	200

Old people living on their own and under poor economic circumstances sometimes show evidence of folate deficiency (Gough *et al.*, 1963; Read *et al.*, 1965). Most workers have measured serum and red cell folate levels (Table 3). Varadi & Elwis (1966) noted that ten out of 81 patients over the age of 70 had reduced red cell folate levels and Elwood *et al.* (1971), in a survey of 533 subjects over the age of 65 in Wales, found that 43 had reduced red cell folate levels – 14 and 8 per cent respectively. In a similar series Hurdle & Picton Williams (1966) found that two out of 71 such patients actually had a megaloblastic process on marrow biopsy.

Assessment on the basis of serum folate levels probably grossly over-estimates the problem. Red cell folate levels suggesting a frequency of 10 per cent probably provide a more realistic estimate of the importance of folate deficiency in the older population. Nevertheless, it is likely that there are marked differences in distribution of folate deficiency throughout different parts of the country as has already been noted in relation to pregnancy; for example, Girdwood, Thomson & Williamson (1967) failed to find any evidence of deficiency in Edinburgh. Often such patients exist on tea and toast as pointed out by Read & co-workers (1965) and are physically disabled or have other illnesses that contribute to their problems.

Folate deficiency is three times as common among Indian immigrants to the UK as compared to Caucasians (Britt *et al.*, 1971).

References

Adams, J. F. & Boddy, K. (1968): *J. Lab. Clin. Med.* 73, 392.

Anderson, B., Belcher, E.H., Chanarin, I. & Mollin, D.L. (1960): *Br. J. Haemat.* 6, 439

Badenoch, J. (1954): *Proc. Roy. Soc. Med.* 47, 426.

Batata, M., Spray, G.H., Bolton, F.G., Higgins, G. & Wollner, L. (1967): *Br. Med. J.* 2, 667.

Bozian, R.C., Ferguson, J.L., Heyssel, R.M., Meneely, G.R. & Darby, W.J. (1963): *Am. J. Clin. Nutr.* **12**, 117.
Britt, R.P., Harper, C. & Spray, G.H. (1971): *Q. Jl Med. N.S.* **40**, 499.
Butterworth, C.E. Jnr., Baugh, C.M. & Krumsieck, C. (1969): *J. Clin. Invest.* **48**, 1131.
Chanarin, I. (1969): *The megaloblastic anaemias*, p. 790. Oxford: Blackwell.
Chanarin, I. (1974): *Getting the most out of food*, No. 10. Burgess Hill: Van den Berghs & Jurgens.
Chanarin, I., Rothamn, D., Ward, A. & Perry, J. (1968): *Br. Med. J.* **2**, 390.
Chanarin, I., Smith, G.V. & Winocour, V. (1969): *Br. J. Haemat.* **16**, 193.
Chung, A.S.M., Pearson, W.N., Darby, W.J., Miller, O.N. & Goldsmith, G.A. (1961): *Am. J. Clin. Nutr.* **9**, 573.
Eichner, E.R., Pierce, H.I. & Hillman, R.S. (1971): *New Engl. J. Med.* **284**, 933.
Ellis, F.R. & Montegriffo, V.M.E. (1970): *Am. J. Clin. Nutr.* **23**, 249.
Elwood, P.C., Shinton, N.K., Wilson, C.I.D., Sweetnam, P. & Frazer, A.C. (1971): *Br. J. Haemat.* **21**, 557.
Estren, S., Brody, E.A. & Wasserman, L.R. (1968): *Adv. Intern. Med.* **9**, 11.
FAO/WHO Expert Group (1970): *Requirements of ascorbic acid, vitamin D, vitamin B_{12} folate and iron.* p. 40. World Health Organisation Tech. Rep. Ser. No. 452: FAO Nutr. Mtgs Rep. Ser. No. 47. Rome: FAO; Geneva: WHO.
Feeley, R.M. & Moyer, E.Z. (1961): *J. Nutr.* **75**, 447.
Ford, J. & Holdsworth, E.S. (1965): Unpublished work. Quoted by Smith, E.L. (1965). *Vitamin B_{12}*, 3rd ed. p. 17. London: Methuen.
Gatenby, P.B.B. (1956): *Proc. Nutr. Soc.* **15**, 115.
Ghitis, J. (1966): *Am. J. Clin. Nutr.* **18**, 452.
Girdwood, R.H., Thomson, A.D. & Williamson, J. (1967): *Br. Med. J.* **2**, 670.
Glass, G.B.J. & Lee, D.H. (1966): *Blood* **27**, 227.
Gough, K.R., Read, A.E. McCarthy, C.F. & Waters, A.H. (1963): *Q.J.Med. N.S.* **32**, 243.
Grasbeck, R. (1960): *Adv. Clin. Chem.* **3**, 299.
Grasbeck. R., Nyberg, W. & Reizenstein, P. (1958): *Proc. Soc. Exp. Biol. Med.* **97**, 780.
Gray, O.P. & Butler, E.B. (1965): *Archs Dis. Childh.* **40**, 53.
Hansen, H. & Rybo, G. (1967): *Acta Obstet. Gynec. Scand.* **46**, Suppl. 7, 107.
Hansen, H.A. & Weinfeld, A. (1962): *Acta. Med. Scand.* **172**, 427.
Heinrich, H.C. (1964): *Seminars in Haematology* **1**, 199.
Herbert, V. (1962*a*): *Trans Ass. Am. Physns* **75**, 307.
Herbert, V. (1962*b*): *Arch. Intern. Med.* **110**, 649.
Heyssel, R.M., Bozian, R.C., Darby, W.J. & Bell, M.C. (1966): *Am. J. Clin. Nutr.* **18**, 176.
Hoffbrand, A.V. (1969): *Br. Med. J.* **1**, 51.
Hurdle, A.D.F. & Picton Williams, T.C. (1966): *Br. Med. J.* **2**, 202.
Jagerstad, M., Lindstrand, K. & Norden, A. (1975*a*): *Scand. J. Soc. Med.* Suppl. 10, 75.
Jagerstad, M., Lindstrand, K. & Westesson, A.-K. (1975*b*): *Scand. J. Soc. Med.* Suppl. 10, 78.
Jolliffe, N & Peterman, R.A. (1956): Folic acid, vitamin B_6, pantothenic acid and vitamin B_{12} in human dietaries. *Am. J. Clin. Nutr.* **9**, 573.
Karlin, R., Hours, C., Bertoye, R., Vallier, C. & Berry, N. (1967): Etude sur les taux d'acide folique de lait humain et du lait bovin. *Int. Z. Vitamin-forsch* **37**, 334.
Lowenstein, L., Cantlie, G., Romas, O. & Brunton, L. (1966): *Can. Med. Ass. J.* **95**, 797.
Matoth, Y., Pinkas, A., Zamir, R., Mooallem, F. & Grossowicz, N. (1964): *Pediatrics* **33**, 507.
Mehta, B.M., Rege, D.V. & Satoskar, R.S. (1964): *Am. J. Clin. Nutr.* **15**, 77.
Moscovitch, L. & Cooper, B.A. (1973): *Am. J. Clin. Nutr.* **26**, 707.
Perry, J. (1971): *Br. J. Haemat.* **21**, 435.
Perry, J. & Chanarin, I. (1968): *Br. Med. J.* **4**, 546.
Read, A.E., Gough, K.R., Pardoe, J.L. & Nicholas, A. (1965): *Br. Med. J.* **2**, 843.
Reizenstein, P.G., Ek, G. & Matthews, C.M.E. (1966): *Phys Med. Biol.* **11**, 295.
Roberts, P.M., Arrowsmith, D.E., Rau, S.M. & Monk-Jones, M.E. (1969): *Archs Dis. Childh.* **44**, 637.
Rosenberg, J.H. & Godwin, H.A. (1971): *Gastroenterology* **60**, 445.
Shojania, A.M. & Gross, S. (1964): *J. Pediat.* **64**, 323.
Smith, A.D.M. (1962): *Brit Med. J.* **1**, 1655.
Stewart, J.S., Roberts, P.D. & Hoffbrand, A.V. (1970): *Lancet* **2**, 542.
Strelling, M.K., Blackledge, G.D., Goodall, H.B. & Walker, C.H.M. (1966): *Lancet* **1**, 898.
Swendseid, M.E., Gasster, M. & Halsted, J.A. (1954): *Proc. Soc. Exp. Biol. Med.* **86**, 834.
Temperley, I.J., Meehan, M.J.M. & Gatenby, P.B.B. (1968): *Br. J. Haemat.* **14**, 13.
Thenen, S.W. (1975): *Am. J. Clin. Nutr.* **22**, 1341.
Toepfer, E.W., Zook, E.G., Orr, M.L. & Richardson, L.R. (1951): *Agriculture handbook No. 29.* US Department of Agriculture.
Vanier, T.M. & Tyas, J.F. (1967): *Archs Dis. Childh.* **42**, 57.
Varadi, S. & Elwis, A. (1966): *Br. Med. J.* **2**, 410.
Zuelzer, W.W. & Ogden, F.N. (1946): *Am. J. Dis. Child.* **71**, 211.

3

Vitamin C: Some unresolved problems

R. E. Hughes.

Introduction

The purpose of this article is not to provide a resume of current knowledge of vitamin C (ascorbic acid, AA) but rather, to highlight those areas which, in the author's opinion, are likely to attract the attention of nutritionists during the next decade.

Hypovitaminosis C and 'extra-antiscorbutic' functions

Scurvy, as classically described (eg Bartley, Krebs & O'Brien, 1953), is today a rare condition in Western Europe. Brook has documented some cases reported in the literature between 1958 and 1972 (Brook, 1972) and since then a few sporadic cases have been reported; we are told that 'manifest clinical scurvy seldom occurs in the United States' (Sauberlich, 1975). The Recommended Daily Intake (RDI) of AA in the United Kingdom (30 mg) was originally derived from the quantity necessary to prevent overt scurvy with a built-in safety factor of three (DHSS, 1969).

Although the mean AA purchased *per capita* is considerably in excess of the RDI yet there is considerable variability in the intake and it has been suggested that up to 10 per cent of households may have an AA intake that is permanently below 30 mg/person per day (Allen, Brook & Broadbent, 1968; Sauberlich, 1975). This situation may be exacerbated by the very considerable losses in AA between purchasing and ingestion (see 'Optimal AA intakes', below).

If one accepts that AA has extra-antiscorbutic functions for which tissue concentrations greater than those necessary to protect against 'overt' scurvy are desirable, then an RDI based on the prevention or cure of frank scurvy becomes less acceptable scientifically and less meaningful nutritionally. Clinical and experimental studies over recent years have certainly suggested that AA probably has a number of such extra-antiscorbutic involvements, ie metabolic involvements distinct from those normally associated with the prevention of classical scurvy (Andrews, 1977; Hughes, 1977). There are, as described below, six reasonably clearly defined areas where the possibility of extra-antiscorbutic functions has been scientifically examined.

(a) Lipid metabolism and atherogenesis
Early observations that cholesterol accumulated in tissues during experimental avitaminosis C (scurvy) stimulated interest in the possible use of AA to modify the concentration and/or distribution of cholesterol and other lipids in the body; this could be of considerable clinical significance as high blood-cholesterol concentrations appear to be a feature of atherogenesis and its clinical sequelae (DHSS Report, 1974). A compound able to reduce blood cholesterol concentrations could be of potential value in the prevention of coronary heart disease. Recent reviews, however, have underlined the highly discrepant results that have emerged in this field, eg in assessing the influence of AA supplementation on plasma triglycerides (Turley, West & Horton, 1976; Ginter, 1978).

Regarding cholesterol itself, two theses have been presented: (1) that AA may modify its endogenous formation, (2) that AA is necessary for its elimination from the body by conversion to bile acids. The evidence for (1) is meagre and debatable; the evidence for (2) is more convincing.

Ginter, on the basis of studies with humans and with 'chronic latent vitamin C deficiency' guinea pigs, has suggested that hypercholesterolaemia is a likely biological consequence of hypovitaminosis C (Hughes, 1976; Ginter, 1978). He has produced evidence that the proper functioning of the enzymic system necessary for the hydroxylytic conversion of cholesterol to bile acids is dependent upon an adequate supply of AA.

If Ginter's hypothesis were correct than one would expect low blood-cholesterol concentrations to be associated with high AA intakes and *vice versa;* this has not always proved to be the case (Elwood, Hughes & Hurley, 1970; Bates, Mandel & Cole, 1977) and in one such population study a *positive* correlation between AA and blood cholesterol was reported (Davies & Newson, 1974).

One should perhaps distinguish between the successful use of large doses of AA to lower blood cholesterol (for which there is little evidence) and the emergence of raised blood cholesterol concentrations in hypovitaminosis C (for which there is some evidence). Ginter's emphasis (Ginter, 1978) is on the preventative aspects of the problem and on the avoidance of hypovitaminosis C rather than on any general pharmacological use of AA as a hypocholesterolaemic agent. Hypercholesterolaemia may presumably result from one or more of a wide range of nutritional and physiological causes. If, in a particular case, hypovitaminosis C is the cause then a response to AA supplementation might be expected. The indiscriminate use of AA megadoses as a supposed hypocholesterolaemic agent in AA-sufficient subjects is, biochemically and nutritionally, a less meaningful exercise.

(b) Cerebral function
There are indications that AA is involved in brain metabolism. Attention has been drawn to a possible relationship between mental depression and AA concentrations (Brook, 1972). There are reports that reduced AA levels result in abnormal patterns in the distribution and biosynthesis of biogenic amines believed to be involved in neural physiology, but it would be difficult to express such changes in terms of cerebral function (Deana *et al.*, 1975; Subramanian, 1977). Pauling quotes studies where mental activity and I.Q. could be correlated with AA intake; he himself has elaborated a system of orthomolecular

psychiatry - the treatment of mental diseases such as schizophrenia by the provision of the optimal molecular environment in the brain - and he attaches considerable importance to large intakes of AA as a means of achieving this state (Pauling, 1976; Hoffer, 1975). To date, orthomolecular theories have made few inroads into orthodox psychiatry (see, eg, Jenner, 1973) and evidence for Pauling's theory that learning and mental acuity could benefit from AA megatherapy is meagre.

Massive doses of AA failed to influence the learning capacity of guinea pigs in a maze (Adlard, Moon & Smart, 1974) - perhaps a not entirely unexpected finding as brain AA is less dependent upon dietary intake than that of other organs and even doses of the order prescribed by megatherapists would be unlikely to produce any substantial shift in the cerebral AA concentration (Hurley, Jones & Hughes, 1972; Spector, 1977).

(c) Protection against infection

Wilson has documented a list of some 30 disease states in which reductions in blood AA concentrations have been reported (Wilson, 1974). Certainly there is evidence that in man leucocyte AA falls during the acute phase of certain diseases (MacLennan & Hamilton, 1977); urinary excretion of AA is changed during experimentally induced infection with common-cold viruses (Davies *et al.*, 1979). Such findings are suggestive of an involvement of AA in infective processes. They do not necessarily mean that AA is likely to have a protective role in infection. Nevertheless, this possibility has attracted the attention of many groups of workers.

Studies have centred on the prevention and/or treatment of the common cold but to make a careful clinical assessment of each subject at each stage of the trial often means that, statistically, an unsatisfactory number of participants has to be used - perhaps as few as 20-30 per group. The alternative is to use as large a number of subjects as possible – say, 100-200 per group – and to rely on subjective evaluations, usually obtained by each subject recording details on a standard-type 'symptoms card'.

Berry & Darke in 1968, in a survey of trials, concluded that 'to date there is no satisfactory evidence that any increase in the present recommended allowance of 30 mg of ascorbic acid is necessary' (Berry & Darke, 1968). Pauling's assessment of more or less the same data was quite different and led him to state that megadoses of AA could reduce both the frequency and severity of colds (Pauling, 1970). More recently, the authors of a comprehensive review in the American Press concluded that their examination of those 'controlled studies ... that meet some reasonable criteria of design reveals little convincing evidence to support claims of clinically important efficacy' (Dykes & Meier, 1975). Pauling, in turn, has produced an expanded version of his original claims (Pauling, 1976).

The reaction of the scientific and medical press to Pauling's claims has, on the whole, been one of benevolent hostility; many have echoed Tyrrell's remark that, in this context, 'belief ... is not evidence' (Tyrrell, 1974). Anderson (1977) in summarizing the results of trials with over 5000 subjects reported that AA supplementation had little effect on the total number of episodes of illness but resulted in a fairly consistent reduction in disability as measured by time spent indoors. He concluded that 'This would seem to indicate that the effect of the vitamin C supplementation is not on a direct local basis on the respiratory organs, or indeed a direct action on the viruses responsible, but rather a more non-specific effect on host resistance, hence the reduction in disability' (Anderson, 1977).

(d) Detoxication

There is considerable evidence that AA may modify the response of the body to toxic substances. There are two main areas of significance in this respect, namely (1) the reduction by AA of the formation and/or toxicity of certain carcinogenic agents and (2) the maintenance at optimal levels of activity of the hepatic microsomal system - the system primarily responsible for the detoxication of foreign substances.

It has been suspected for some years that AA offers protection against certain chemically-induced growths. The use of supplemental doses of AA to prevent the formation of bladder tumours induced by 3-hydroxy anthranilic acid is probably one of the best documented examples (Schlegel *et al.*, 1970). But the role of AA in the formation/carcinogenicity of the nitrosamines is probably the system that has received most attention.

Animal studies have indicated that N-nitrosamines are carcinogenic, although their exact significance in humans has yet to be established. Nitrosamines may be formed wherever nitrate, a suitable nitrosable amine and bacteria co-exist. The nitrate is first converted by bacterial action to nitrite which then reacts with amines to produce the carcinogenic nitrosamines; epidemiological studies point to a high incidence of gastric cancer in areas where nitrate intake is high (Wolff & Wasserman, 1972; Hill, 1980).

There is evidence that this formation of nitrosoamines can be blocked by AA (Mirvish *et al.*, 1972; Kamm *et al.*, 1973). Weisburger has emphasised the protective role that additive AA could have in this context; he and his colleagues have shown that a fish eaten in Japan, where the incidence of gastric cancer is high, yielded a mutagen when treated with nitrite, but not in the presence of AA (Weisburger, 1977; Marquardt, Rufino & Weisburger, 1977).

Recent evidence has suggested that AA may inhibit not only the formation of nitrosamines but also their mutagenicity. Correa, Kikatnur & Murray (1978) have suggested that spermidine may be the critical precursor amine for nitroso formation in gastric cancer and they have reported that its mutagenicity was reduced by AA whether it was added before or after the nitrosamine formation. Hill, in reminding us of the speculation that endogenously produced N-nitroso compounds may be the 'universal initiator' in human carcinogenesis, has indicated that there may now be a case for initiating clinical trials to study the value of AA supplementation in the prevention of carcinogenesis. This, he implies, could be of especial value in areas where there are indications of a possible nitrosamine involvement in the causative phase such as in gastric cancer or after certain surgical manipulations where the urinary flow (including its bacterial flora) is diverted into the colon (Hill, 1980).

The evidence that AA has a role in the hepatic microsomal system stems, for the most part, from studies on deficient or hypovitaminotic-C guinea pigs. There would appear to be fairly general agreement that low tissue concentrations of AA in guinea pigs result in a reduced detoxication capacity, involving both microsomal hydroxylation and demethylation systems, and associated electron transport components, such as cytochrome P-450 (Degwitz & Staudinger, 1974; Fielding & Hughes, 1975; Zannoni & Sato, 1976). The main findings have been usefully summarised recently (Zannoni, Sato & Rikans, 1978).

A significant feature of these findings is that the depressed hepatic metabolism of drugs frequently emerged well before the more generally accepted signs of scurvy in guinea pigs (Conney *et al.*, 1961; Zannoni, Flynn & Lynch, 1972; Street & Chadwick, 1975). Parke (1978), in a corollary to this type of study, has reported that the long-term administration of chlordiazepoxide (Librium) to guinea pigs and humans increased the need for AA - presumably because of its probable involvement in the metabolism of the drug.

The exact relevance of these animal detoxication studies to human nutrition is not known. Of possible interest are reports that the microsomal drug metabolising enzymes and their induction are depressed in elderly men (Bender, 1964; Vestal *et al.* 1975, Salem *et al.*, 1978). This could be an example of the well documented changes in enzyme activity with age; on the other hand, it could reflect the low AA concentrations generally characteristic of 'old' tissues (see below 'Ascorbic acid and ageing'). Certainly further studies of drug metabolism in man *vis-a-vis* AA status could produce useful information.

(e) Cancer

Recent claims of a role for AA in cancer therapy have attracted much attention but little scientific support. The protagonists of the theory have recently presented their main arguments plausibly, if not fully convincingly, in a well documented article (Cameron, Pauling & Leibovitz, 1979). In their earlier paper Cameron & Pauling (1976) reported that AA megadoses (about 10 g daily) quadrupled the survival time of terminal cancer patients; 100 such patients were given AA megadoses and their survival time compared with 1000 controls - ie ten matched controls for each treated patient. The overall difference between the survival times of the two groups was of a high order of statistical significance. The authors' most recent conclusion is that:

'Present evidence suggests to us that supplemental ascorbate can offer some degree of benefit to all advanced cancer patients and quite remarkable benefit to a fortunate few and it has even greater potential value in the supportive treatment of earlier and more favourable patients' (Cameron, Pauling & Leibovitz, 1979).

The almost calculated indifference which the scientific press has accorded these claims is perhaps unfortunate. Certainly a carefully controlled clinical trial would be not inappropriate and would do much to resolve the doubts of non-clinical nutritionists and pharmacologists (for this is not, in essence, a nutritional problem at all). As matters stand, there is no evidence that AA retards the growth of tumours in guinea pigs (Migliozzi, 1977), nor does it enhance the immune response or the formation of PHI (physiological hyaluronidase inhibitor) - two systems whose activities are central to the Cameron-Pauling hypothesis (Kalden & Guthy, 1972).

(f) Fatigue

A 'listlessness to action' and an aversion to any sort of exercise... soon degenerating into a universal lassitude and much fatigue' was a first indication of the approach of scurvy according to Lind (1753). Studies with human volunteers have confirmed that lassitude and fatigue precede the emergence of the more clearly definable clinical features of scurvy (van Eekelen, 1936; Crandon *et al.*, 1940; Hodges *et al.*, 1971). The recent finding that AA is a co-factor for the conversion of lysine to carnitine (Hulse *et al.*, 1978) provides a link between hypovitaminosis C and physical fatigue. Carnitine (β-OH-γ [trimethylamino] butyric acid) has a biochemical role as a carrier molecule for the transport of fatty acid residues into the mitochondria where they may be oxidized (Bremer, 1977). By modifying the availability of muscle fatty acid for energy production carnitine may thereby influence the capacity of the muscle to maintain sustained contraction. Muscle weakness and fatigue are common features of clinical carnitine deficiency (Karpati *et al.*, 1975) and recent studies have shown that in guinea-pigs a restricted AA intake results in a significant fall in muscle carnitine *before* the emergence of any of the symptoms customarily regarded as characteristic of scurvy (Hughes, Hurley & Jones, 1980). Muscle carnitine, in the guinea-pig, may therefore serve as a highly sensitive indicator of AA status. Currrent thought on the RDI for AA derives primarily from a consideration of the amount of the vitamin required to prevent the emergence of 'clinical' scurvy. Because of this, the carnitine-fatigue-AA relationship would appear to merit further study: the existence in man of a relationship similar to that in the guinea-pig would be a strong reason for re-appraising current thought on the optimal intake of the vitamin.

Resolution of the 'extra-antiscorbutic' claims remains one of the main problems of current nutrition. Two general points may be made. First, it may well emerge that in the final analysis they may all be shown to be variations on a basic hydroxylation theme. A collagen-like amino acid sequence is a characteristic of other structures in the body such as the $C1_q$ complement subcomponent (Porter, 1977) and the basement membrane (Kefalides, 1973) and some of the postulated 'extra-antiscorbutic' involvements may be resolved in terms not entirely unrelated to the currently accepted biochemical explanation of the mode of action of AA in preventing scurvy. Certainly a hydroxylation mechanism would appear to be central to the probable role of AA in cholesterol metabolism, in some detoxication mechanisms and in the fatigue-carnitine relationship. Second, it may be noted that there is accumulating evidence that the requirement of AA for the extra-antiscorbutic aspects is probably greater than that required for the prevention of overt scurvy - a significant point in terms of recommended daily intakes.

Optimal intakes of ascorbic acid

In the present state of knowledge it is meaningless to speak of an optimum level for dietary AA as we have no means of relating AA intake to the supposed extra-antiscorbutic functions. All that is known is that in a number of cases the requirement is greater than that necessary to prevent the emergence of overt clinical scurvy. It would not appear to be unreasonable in the circumstances to suggest that tissue saturation or near-saturation with AA should be regarded as a physiologically-desirable goal. This would prevent the emergence of any pre- or sub-scorbutic changes and would appear to be a more meaningful aim for compilers of 'healthful' diet recommendations than the mere prevention of arbitrarily selected 'overt' symptoms.

The intake of AA necessary to attain tissue saturation has been for some years a matter of debate. Early studies, based essentially on the response of blood and urine to graded intakes of AA, indicated that a sustained daily intake of 60-100 mg would achieve tissue saturation (Irwin & Hutchins, 1976). Recent work has confirmed this. In adult females a daily intake of 140 mg produced essentially the same concentration of leucocyte AA as a daily 'megadose' of 1 g (R.E. Hughes *et al.*, Unpublished). Studies with labelled AA indicated that 45 mg AA daily would maintain the body pool at 'maximum saturation' (Hodges *et al.*, 1971; Baker *et al.*, 1971). More recently, Kallner, Hartmann & Hornig (1979) using similar techniques have concluded that a total turnover of c. 60 mg/day should be aimed at; correcting for incomplete absorption, this should equal c. 70-75 mg/day, which, on adding 2 x s.d. to reach 95 per cent of the population, would suggest a daily intake of c. 100 mg.

There are, of course, certain important qualifications to any generalisations about the relationship between dietary AA and tissue concentrations, as follows.

(a) One should be aware of the considerable discrepancy, in most populations, between AA *purchased* and AA *ingested*. Dietary surveys do not in general relate to the amounts of AA actually ingested and they frequently ignore the very considerable losses of AA that occur during the processing and domestic preparation of foods. Surprisingly low AA intakes have been reported where the actual analyses have been done on the food samples immediately before ingestion (Disselduff & Murphy, 1968; Burr *et al.*, 1974*b*).

This discrepancy between 'nutrient purchased' and 'nutrient ingested' is probably far greater for AA than for any other nutrient; dietary surveys based on actual analyses of 'ingested AA' would appear to be long overdue - particularly perhaps amongst disadvantaged and anomalous sectors of the population such as the institutionalised elderly (Andrews, 1973). Further, variable, losses in AA probably occur during passage through and absorption from, the gastrointestinal tract. To provide a daily intake of 50-100 mg the 'AA purchased' should be substantially greater than this.

(b) In certain anomalous sectors of the population — either because of greater metabolic demand for AA or because of its increased destruction by and/or loss from the body — the daily requirement for the vitamin could be in excess of the normal range. Thus it is officially recommended that during pregnancy and lactation the intake of AA be increased from 30 to 60 mg (DHSS, 1979). Smoking, slimming, contraceptive agents, dietary bioflavonoids and many other factors have been shown to influence tissue AA levels — usually by reducing its concentration (Pelletier, 1975; Davies & Hughes, 1977; Rivers, 1975; Hughes & Wilson, 1977). Whether these effects represent specific metabolic happenings or whether they merely reflect a general lability on the part of tissue AA is not known. There is a tendency however to assume that any circumstance resulting in a lowered tissue (or blood) AA concentration calls for a corresponding increase in the intake.

In specifying AA optimal requirements one should perhaps not discount the influence of biochemical individuality. There are indications that biochemical individuality with respect to AA, previously commented on in guinea pigs (Williams & Deacon, 1967), extends also to man (Yew, 1975). The anomalous subject, whose blood AA in no way reflects his dietary intake of the vitamin, is a familiar feature of many nutritional surveys and underlines the significance of individual idiosyncracies in absorption and/or metabolism.

Hypervitaminosis C and AA 'megatherapy'

The arguments for AA megatherapy (the ingestion of massive doses of the vitamin) were first outlined by Irwin Stone and later re-presented and elaborated by Linus Pauling. Stone's original thesis appeared in a number of speculative papers published between 1965 and 1967 (Stone, 1965; 1966*a,b*; 1967) Stone regarded the recommended daily intakes for AA as grossly inadequate. He based his argument primarily on a consideration of those species able to synthesise their own AA; some four or five species, including man, are known to have lost this ability to produce AA endogenously and are perforce dependent upon dietary sources of the vitamin. Stone pointed out that animals producing their own AA do so at a comparatively high rate; per 70 kg body weight (the weight of an average man) the daily production would be 1.8 g (rat), 15.8 g (rabbit) and 19.3 g (mouse).

Man's daily intake, according to Stone, should therefore be of this order to restore the nutritional *status quo* existing before he lost his capacity to produce AA. An integral feature of Stone's argument is the assumption that organisms always synthesise metabolites at an optimal rate; this would be challenged by many biochemists and particularly perhaps by clinicians striving to depress tissue levels of endogenously produced cholesterol and oxalic acid.

Stone also quotes, with approval, Bourne's estimate that the natural diet of the gorilla provides it with a daily intake of some 4.5 g AA (Bourne, 1949) and this, he argues, should be taken as an index to man's 'natural requirement'. Pauling has developed this argument by calculating that if man ate a 'natural' diet of nuts, grains, fruit and vegetables his AA intake would be about 2.3 g/day - some 80 times the current RDI in the UK (Pauling, 1976). Jukes (1974) has criticised Pauling's calculations on two counts: (1) that Pauling's 'natural diet' contained horticultural innovations that would have been absent from primitive man's dietary pattern and (2) that the comparatively high intake of AA by primitive man was fortuitous and of no especial nutritional significance. As Jukes points out 'If an animal is consuming a mixture of plant foods to satisfy the need for calories, the non-caloric ingredients will be ingested at levels that do not necessarily correspond to a quantitative nutritional requirement' (Jukes, 1974). Juke's point is a valid one; 'natural diets' contained comparatively high amounts of phytic acid, organic acids, alkaloids etc but it would be difficult to substantiate a claim that the 'natural' intake of these substances represented a nutritionally-optimal level.

Nevertheless, there are probably some hundreds of thousands of megatherapists of varying degrees in the United Kingdom, consuming between them annually some tons of AA. From time to time fears have been expressed about the possible disadvantages of sustained AA megatherapy, although the actual number of cases where an apparent adverse effect has been clearly demonstrated are few (Goldstein, 1971; Jackish, 1971; Horrobin, 1973; Schrauzer & Rhead, 1973; Campbell, Steinberg & Bower, 1975; Mengel & Greene, 1976). On the other hand, a number of workers have been unable to detect any untoward effects in patients given megadoses of AA over comparatively long periods (eg Hoffer, 1971).

In more general terms, theoretical considerations of the possible disadvantages of AA megatherapy have centred on these areas:

(1) Increased susceptibility to scurvy on cessation of AA megatherapy. It has been reasoned that the overall AA metabolism of the body becomes geared to high intakes of AA and that an abrupt cessation of megatherapy may precipitate a condition of AA deficiency. This is the thesis presented by Rhead & Shrauzer (1971) who referred to individual cases where scorbutic symptoms emerged on cessation of AA megadosing. These workers later reported that the blood AA levels of subjects who had received AA megadoses (1-3 g daily for periods of up to 54 months) fell to below-control values on cessation of dosing, a finding also reported by Masek & Hruba (Masek & Hruba, 1969, 1974; Schrauzer & Rhead, 1973). Complementary studies with guinea pigs have, however, given conflicting results (Gordonoff, 1960; Hornig *et al.*, 1973; Nandi *et al.*, 1973; Sorensen, Devine & Rivers, 1974). Cochrane, in discussing systemic conditioning in the context of prenatal and neonatal nutrition, has suggested that infantile scurvy could be a consequence of *in utero* exposure to maternal megatherapy (Cochrane, 1965).

(2) Increased formation and excretion of oxalic acid. Oxalic acid is an end-product of AA metabolism in man and the influence of increased AA intakes on oxalic acid excretion has received some attention. It is assumed that any substantial increase in oxalic acid formation could further renal calcification and the formation of calculi. On balance, it would appear that fairly substantial intakes of AA (4-9 g daily) are necessary to produce any significant change in the urinary excretion of oxalic acid (Lamden & Chrystowski, 1954; Wyngaarden & Elder, 1966), although a recent study has indicated that a daily intake of 1 g AA by adult females produced a significantly greater output of oxalic acid than a daily supplement of orange juice containing 100 mg AA (R.E. Hughes *et al.* Unpublished).

The significance of these findings is, however, somewhat obscure as there is no general agreement on how much urinary oxalate is physiologically acceptable. It has been suggested that even a comparatively small increase in oxalic acid excretion could disadvantage a person 'with a high normal or elevated level of urinary oxalate' (Smith, 1972). Increases in oxalate formation should, of course, always be considered in relation to the body calcium status. In adults, a high urinary oxalate in the presence of elevated calcium levels could enhance the formation of calcium oxalate which, because of its limited solubility in urine, could increase any tendency to stone formation; in young, growing subjects with a marginal or non-optimal calcium intake, excess oxalate formation could modify the availability of calcium.

Briggs (1976) reported that out of 67 screened by him for AA-induced hyperoxaluria three (including a father and his son) excreted greatly increased amounts of oxalic acid (600-700 mg daily) after ingesting 4 g AA daily for 7 days. AA-induced hyperoxaluria of this order could well be regarded as a contra-indication for AA megatherapy – always assuming, of course, that the oxalic acid is not being produced in place of other, more toxic metabolites.

(3) Increased toxicity of metals. There is evidence that increased intakes of AA enhance the absorption of certain metals from the gastrointestinal tract (Hughes, 1974). The physiological significance of this type of relationship depends upon the nature of the metal involved. In the case of iron it is usually regarded as a beneficial one; but any AA enhancement of the uptake of a toxic metal can only disadvantage the body. It has been reported that AA megadoses given to guinea pigs exposed to dietary mercury doubled the deposition of mercury in the tissues and halved the survival time of the guinea pigs (Blackstone, Hurley & Hughes, 1974; Murray & Hughes, 1976).

It would be of interest to determine (a) whether AA enhances the passage of mercury across other biological membranes and (b) whether the membrane transport of other toxic metals, such as cadmium and lead, is influenced in a similar way. The influence of *in utero* exposure to maternal megatherapy on the uptake of toxic metals by the foetal brain could also be of some significance in this context.

(4) Possible toxicity of AA breakdown products. Knowledge of the catabolism of AA in the tissues is incomplete and little is known of the nature and metabolic significance, if any, of the products of its metabolism. Neither the monkey nor guinea pigs can be used as models for human catabolic studies as the pathways of AA metabolism are different in the three species (King & Burns, 1975; Lewin, 1976).

Still less is known about the nature and metabolic significance of the products resulting from the chemical breakdown of AA. This is surprising when one considers that comparatively large amounts of AA are used industrially as a permitted additive under conditions which result in the formation of a considerable range of breakdown products. In the United States alone the annual production of ascorbate probably exceeds ten million kilograms (Ginter, 1979). It has been estimated that about half of the AA produced synthetically is used in the food industry, the bulk of it as a technological aid, the main areas of application being the soft drinks industry, in meat curing and pickling, in the fermentation industries and to improve the baking quality of flour (Klaui, 1974).

In the baking industry the additive AA is almost completely broken down during processing; Thewlis (1974) has shown that 87 per cent of the original AA could be accounted for as CO_2 (24 per cent), L-threonic acid (52 per cent) and 2,3-diketogulonic acid (11 per cent). Other breakdown products have been characterised in different systems; one group of workers isolated as many as 15 products from the *in vitro* breakdown of AA (Tatum, Shaw & Berry, 1969). The average consumer will probably ingest daily some tens of milligrammes of a number of AA breakdown products whose metabolism and physiological significance are far from clearly defined.

Of relevance in this context are reports that breakdown products of AA, formed by incubating the AA with cupric ions, are mutagenic in bacterial and animal cells (Stich *et al.*, 1976; Omura *et al.*, 1978). It is widely accepted that the majority of carcinogenic agents are mutagens (Paget, 1979); mutagens are possibly of significance too in the ageing processes (Burnet, 1976). Factors which modify the formation of mutagenic breakdown products from AA could therefore be of some physiological significance.

Nor can AA breakdown products be considered in isolation from megatherapy practices as any increase in the AA intake will presumably result in the formation of greater amounts of breakdown products particularly in the gastrointestinal tract. The absorption of single megadoses of AA is a relatively inefficient process with a comparatively rapid saturation of the intestinal transport mechanism (Kubler & Gehler, 1970; Mayersohn, 1972; Nelson *et al.*, 1978). In the normal adult over 50 per cent of a 1 g megadose passes through the gastrointestinal tract unabsorbed and with a 5 g dose the absorption may be as low as 25 per cent (R.E. Hughes & E. Jones, Unpublished).

Much of the unabsorbed AA will presumably undergo breakdown (both chemical and bacterial) in the intestinal tract to produce a whole range of compounds whose influence on the tissues is almost completely unknown. The formation of such compounds will in turn be influenced by factors such as the gastrointestinal pH and the rate of movement of the intestinal contents. Their accumulation in the gastrointestinal tract, or in the tissues after absorption, could elicit somatic changes with possible pathogenic consequences.

A study of the nutritional significance of AA breakdown products and metabolites would appear to be one of the more demanding problems of nutritional science. In the meantime, persons wishing to supplement their daily intake of AA should perhaps consider (1) taking their supplement as a fruit juice preparation the flavonoid content of which would to some extent retard the breakdown of AA during ingestion and the passage of AA along the gastrointestinal tract (Hughes & Wilson, 1977); (2) limiting their daily supplement to the amount necessary to attain tissue saturation.

Ascorbic acid and ageing

The relationship between AA and the ageing process(es) has attracted attention for some time. A negative correlation between age and blood AA exists in man (eg Kirk & Chieffi, 1953; Andrews & Brook, 1966) and between age and tissue AA concentrations in guinea pigs (Hughes & Jones, 1971). Lewin has usefully summarised results for human tissues of different ages (Lewin, 1976). A number of factors may contribute to a relationship of this kind, namely: (1) a lowered AA intake, (2) a reduced gastrointestinal absorption, (3) a reduced renal threshold, (4) an increased metabolic demand for AA, (5) a reduced tissue capacity to conserve/retain AA.

Some have interpreted the low AA concentrations in elderly subjects as indicative of a state of deficiency and have sought to correlate certain features of ill-health in the elderly with low AA concentrations (eg Griffiths, 1968; Taylor, 1968). However, it is now believed that some of the lesions previously described in this context are non-specific of AA deficiency (Andrews & Brook, 1966;

Andrews, 1977). Until we attain a more extensive knowledge of the AA requirement of elderly subjects we cannot meaningfully interpret low AA levels in the elderly as representing a state of deficiency. The AA requirement and metabolism of old tissues may be quite different from those of younger members of the same species.

There are, for example, grounds for believing that 'old' tissues have a reduced capacity for retaining AA and the negative correlation between AA and age could merely be a reflection of this (Williams & Hughes, 1972; Hughes, 1973). Recent work has supported this theory. It has been shown that saturation levels of old tissues are significantly lower than those of young ones (Davies, Pulsinelli & Hughes, 1976). Again, in elderly subjects (a substantial proportion of whom had serum AA concentrations below 0.2 mg/100 ml) no correlation could be established between morbidity indices and blood AA concentrations (Burr *et al.*, 1974*a*). Attempts to raise the AA concentrations of elderly subjects to those of younger ones could therefore be methodologically difficult and physiologically unrewarding.

Perhaps more attention should be given to the categorisation of population groups with respect to tissue AA concentrations and dietary requirements; it is scientifically unsatisfactory to assess a group's AA status in terms of the established pattern within a quite different group. This, as indicated above, is important where the groups are differentiated in terms of age - but other differentiating factors such as diet, occupation, environment or geographical location could be equally important. The significance of a recent report quoting, for a clearly definable group, unusually low values for normal blood AA levels seems to have escaped the attention of most nutritionists (Davies & Newson, 1974).

The considerable biochemical versatility of the ascorbic acid molecule (Lewin, 1976) could also imply a direct effect on ageing itself. In Pauling's view (1976) sustained AA megatherapy could extend one's life span by as much as 18 years. A sustained state of tissue saturation with respect to AA could influence the GSH:GSSG ratio, of possible significance in ageing changes (Tas, 1976). A further possibility is that ascorbic acid, as a scavenger of toxic radicals such as the superoxide radical O_2^-, may reduce the incidence of deleterious changes of the type implicit to any somatic mutation theory of ageing (Granich, 1972; Hayaishi & Asada, 1977). There is some evidence that antioxidants such as AA prolong the life span of experimental animals (Emanuel *et al.*, 1977).

However, mortality studies in elderly humans have produced no evidence that AA supplementation prolongs the life span (Burr, Hurley & Sweetnam, 1975; Wilson, 1973); both in *Drosophila melanogaster* and the guinea pig, AA supplementation at high dietary concentrations appeared to shorten the life span (Massie, Baird & Piekielniak, 1976; Davies, Ellery & Hughes, 1977) and high tissue AA concentrations did not produce any measurable reduction of lipofuscin - the 'ageing pigment' - in guinea pigs (Ellery, Hughes & Jones, 1979).

Conclusions

Future studies on vitamin C will probably centre on its possible role in areas other than the prevention of 'classical' scurvy. It is probable that the optimal requirement of vitamin C for such 'extra-antiscorbutic' involvements is greater than the current recommended daily amount. The maintenance of tissue saturation (or near saturation) with vitamin C could therefore become a desirable aim. Saturation may be achieved with daily doses of 100-150 mg vitamin C.

Arguments in favour of much larger doses (megatherapy) do not receive general acceptance; there are reasons for believing that AA megatherapy may even be physiologically damaging to the body.

References

Adlard, B.P.F., Moon, S. & Smart, J.L. (1974): *Nature* 247, 398.

Allen, R.J.L., Brook, M. & Broadbent, S.R. (1968): *Br. J. Nutr.* 22, 555.

Anderson, T.W. (1977): *Acta Vit. Enzymol.* 31, 43.

Andrews, J. (1973): *Geront. Clin.* 15, 221.

Andrews, J. (1977): *Proc. Roy. Soc. Med.* 70, 84.

Andrews, J. & Brook, M. (1966): *Lancet* 1, 1350.

Baker, E.M., Hammer, D.G., March, S.C., Tolbert, B.M. & Canham, J.E. (1971): *Science* 173, 826.

Bartley, W., Krebs, H.A. & O'Brien, J.R.P. (1953): *Med. Res. Counc. Spec. Rep. Ser. No. 280.* London: HMSO.

Bates, C.J., Mandel, A.R. & Cole, T.J. (1977): *Lancet* 2, 611.

Bender, A.D. (1964): *J. Am. Geriatr. Soc.* 12, 114.

Berry, W.T.C. & Darke, S.J. (1968): *Practitioner* 201, 305.

Blackstone, S., Hurley, R.J. & Hughes, R.E. (1974): *Fd Cosmet. Toxicol.* 12, 511.

Bourne, G. (1949): *Br. J. Nutr.* 2, 346.

Bremer, J. (1977): *Trends Biochem. Sci.* 2, 207.

Briggs, M.H. (1976): *Lancet* 1, 154.

Brook, M. (1972): In *Nutritional deficiencies in modern society* ed A.N. Howard & I.M. Baird, p. 45. London: Newman Books.

Burnet, F.M. (1976): *Immunology, ageing and cancer.* San Francisco: Freeman.

Burr, M.L., Elwood, P.C., Hole, D.J., Hurley, R.J. & Hughes, R.E. (1974*a*): *Am. J. Clin. Nutr.* 27, 144.

Burr, M.L., Sweetnam, P.M., Hurley, R.J. & Powell, G.H. (1974*b*): *Lancet* 1, 162.

Burr, M.L., Hurley, R.J. & Sweetnam, P.M. (1975): *Geront. Clin.* 17, 236.

Cameron, W. & Pauling, L. (1976): *Proc. Natl. Acad. Sci. USA.* 73, 3685.

Cameron, E., Pauling, L. & Leibovitz, B. (1979): *Cancer Res.* 39, 663.

Campbell, G.D., Steinberg, M.H. & Bower, J.D. (1975): *Ann. Intern. Med.* 82, 810.

Cochrane, W.A. (1965): *Can; Med. Assoc. J.* 93, 893.

Conney, A.H., Bray, G.A., Evans, C. & Burns, J.J. (1961): *Ann. N.Y. Acad. Sci.* 92, 115.

Correa, P., Kokatnur, M.G. & Murray, M.L. (1978): *Lancet* 1, 324.

Crandon, J.H., Lund, M.D. & Dill, D.B. (1940): *N. Eng. J. Med.* 223, 353.

Davies, J.D.G. & Newson, J. (1974): *Am. J. Clin. Nutr.* 27, 1039.

Davies, J.E.W. & Hughes, R.E. (1977): *Br. J. Nutr.* 38, 299.

Davies, J.E.W., Pulsinelli, J. & Hughes, R.E. (1976): *Proc. Nutr. Soc.* 35, 117A.

Davies, J.E.W., Ellery, P.M. & Hughes, R.E. (1977): *Exp. Geront.* 12, 215.

Davies, J.E.W., Hughes, R.E., Jones, R., Reed, S.E., Craig, J.W. & Tyrell, D.A.J. (1979): *Biochem. Med.* 21, 78.

Deana, R., Bjaraj, B.S., Verjee, Z.H. & Galzigna, L. (1975): *J. Vit. Res.* 45, *175.*

Degkwitz, E. & Staudinger, Hj. (1974): In *'Vitamin C'* ed G.G. Birch & K. Parker, p. 161. London: Applied Science Publishers.

DHSS (1969): *Recommended intakes of nutrients for the United Kingdom.* Rep. Publ. Hlth Med. Subj. No. 120. London: HMSO. (see also, DHSS 1979: *Recommended daily amounts of food energy and nutrients for groups of people in the United Kingdom.* Rep. Hlth Soc. Subj. No. 15. London: HMSO).

DHSS (1974): *Diet and coronary heart disease.* London: HMSO.

Disselduff, M.M. & Murphy, E. La. C. (1968): In *Vitamins in the elderly,* ed A.N. Exton-Smith & D.L. Scott, p. 60. Bristol: Wright.
Dykes, M.H.M. & Meier, P. (1975): *J. Am. Med. Ass.* **231**, 1073.
Ellery, P.M., Hughes, R.E. & Jones, E. (1979): *Exp. Gerontol.* **14**, 49.
Elwood, P.C., Hughes, R.E. & Hurley, R.J. (1970): *Lancet* **1**, 1197.
Emanuel, N.N., Obukhova, L.K., Smirnov, L.D. & Bunto, T.V. (1977): *Biol. Bull. Acad. Sci. USSR* (English translation) **4**, 10.
Fielding, A.M. & Hughes, R.E. (1975): *Experientia* **31**, 1394.
Ginter, E. (1978): *Adv. Lipid Res.* **16**, 167.
Ginter, E. (1979): *Am. J. Clin. Nutr,* **32**, 511.
Goldstein, M.L. (1971): *J. Am. Med. Ass.* **216**, 332.
Gordonoff, T. (1960): *Scheiz. Med. Wschr.* **90**, 726.
Granich, M. (1972): In *Developmental physiology and ageing,* ed P.S. Timiras, p. 607. New York: MacMillan.
Griffiths, L.L. (1968): In *Vitamins in the elderly,* ed A.N. Exton-Smith & D.L. Scott. Bristol: Wright.
Hill, M.J. (1980): *Br. Med. Bull.* **36**, 89.
Hayaishi, O. & Asada, K. (1977): *Biochemical and medical aspects of active oxygen.* Baltimore: University Park Press.
Hodges, R.E., Hood, J., Canham, J.E., Sauberlich, H.E. & Baker, E.M. (1971): *Am. J. Clin. Nutr.* **24**, 432.
Hoffer, A. (1971): *New. Engl. J. Med.* **285**, 635.
Hoffer, A. (1975): *Impact Sci. Soc.* **25**, 3.
Hornig, D., Weiser. H., Weber, F. & Wiss, O. (1973): *Int. Z. Vitamin. Forsch.* **43**, 28.
Horrobin, D.F. (1973): *Lancet* **2**, 317.
Hughes, R.E. (1973): *Proc. Nutr. Soc.* **32**, 243.
Hughes, R.E. (1974): In *Vitamin C,* ed G.G. Birch & K.J. Parker, p. 68. London: Applied Science Publishers.
Hughes, R.E. (1976): *J. Hum. Nutr.* **30**, 315.
Hughes, R.E. (1977): *Proc. Roy. Soc. Med.* **70**, 86.
Hughes, R.E. & Jones, P.R. (1971): *Br. J. Nutr.* **25**, 77.
Hughes, R.E. & Wilson, H.K. (1977): *Progr. Med. Chem.* **14**, 285.
Hughes, R.E., Hurley, R.J. & Jones, Eleri (1980): *Br. J. Nutr.* **43**, 385.
Hulse, J.D., Ellis, S.R. & Henderson, L.M. (1978): *J. Biol. Chem.* **253**, 1654.
Hurley, R.J., Jones, P.R. & Hughes, R.E. (1972): *Nutr. Metab.* **14**, 136.
Irwin, M.I. & Hutchins, B.K. (1976): *J. Nutr.* **106**, 821.
Kackisch, P.F. (1971): *Chem. Eng. News* **49**, 86.
Jenner, F.A. (1973): *Lancet* **2**, 787.
Jukes, T.H. (1974): *Proc. Nat. Acad. Sci. USA.* **71**, 1949.
Kalden, J.R. & Guthy, E.A. (1972): *Eur. Surg. Res.* **4**, 114.
Kallner, A., Hartmann, D. & Hornig, D. (1979): *Am. J. Clin. Nutr.* **32**, 530.
Kamm, J.J., Dashman, T., Conney, A.H. & Barns, J.H. (1973): *Proc. Nat. Acad. Sci. USA* **70**, 747.
Karpati, G., Carpenter, S., Engel, A.G. *et al.* (1975): *Neurology* **25**, 16.
Kefalides, N.A. (1973): *Int. Rev. Conn. Tiss. Res.* **6**, 63.
King, C.G. & Burns, J.J. (1975): *Ann. N.Y. Acad, Sci.* 255.
Kirk, J.E. & Chieffi, M. (1953): *J. Gerontol.* **8**, 301.
Klaui, H. (1974): In *Vitamin C,* ed C.G. Birch & K. Parker, p. 16. London: Applied Science Publishers.
Kubler, W. & Gehler, J. (1970): *Int. Z. Vit. Forschung.* **40**, 442.
Lamden, M.P. & Chrystowski, G.A. (1954): *Proc. Soc. Exp. Biol. Med.* **85**, 190.
Lewin, S. (1976): *Vitamin C: its molecular biology and medical potential.* New York: Academic Press.
Lind, J. (1753): *'A treatise of the scurvy'*, p. 148. Edinburgh, London: A. Millar.
MacLennan, W.J. & Hamilton, J.C. (1977): *Br. J. Nutr.* **38**, 217.
Marquardt, H., Rufino, F. & Weisburger, J.H. (1977): *Fd Cosmet. Toxicol.* **15**, 37.

Masek, J. & Hruba, F. (1969): *Int. J. Vit. Res.* **34**, 39.
Masek, J. & Hruba, F. (1974): *Vnitrni Lek* **20**, 670.
Massie, H.R., Baird, M.B. & Piekielniak, M.J. (1976): *Exp. Geront.* **11**, 37.
Mayersohn, M. (1972): *Europ. J. Pharmacol.* **19**, 140.
Mengel, C.E. & Greene, H.L. (1976): *Ann. Intern. Med.* **84**, 490.
Migliozzi, J.A. (1977): *Br. J. Cancer* **35**, 448.
Mirvish, S.S., Wallcave, L., Eagen, M. & Shubik, P. (1972): *Science,* **177**, 65.
Murray, D.R. & Hughes, R.E, (1976): *Proc. Nutr. Soc.* **35**, 118A.
Nandi, B.K., Majumder, A.K., Subramanian, N. & Chatterjee, I.B. (1973): *J. Nutr.* **103**, 1688.
Nelson, E.W., Lane, H., Fabri, P.J. & Scott, B. (1978): *J. Clin. Pharmacol.* **18**, 325.
Omura, H., Shinohara, K., Maeda, H., Nonaka, M. & Murakami, H. (1978): *J. Nutr. Sci. Vitaminol.* **24**, 185.
Paget, G.E., editor (1979): *Mutagenesis in sub-mammalian systems.* Lancaster: MTP Press.
Parke, D.V. (1978): *Wld Rev. Nutr. Diet.* **29**, 96.
Pauling, L. (1970): *Vitamin C and the common cold.* New York: Freeman.
Pauling, L. (1976): *Vitamin C, the common cold and the flu.* San Francisco: Freeman.
Pelletier, O. (1975): *Ann. N.Y. Acad. Sci.* **258**, 156.
Porter, R.R. (1977): *Biochem. Soc. Trans.* **5**, 1659.
Rhead, W.J. & Schrauzer, G.N. (1971): *Nutr. Rev.* **29**, 262.
Rivers, J.M. (1975): *Am. J. Clin. Nutr.* **28**, 550.
Salem, S.A.M., Rajjayabun, P., Shepherd, A.M.M. & Stevenson, I.H. (1978): *Age & Ageing* **7**, 68.
Sauberlich, H.E. (1975): *Ann. N.Y. Acad. Sci.* **258**, 438.
Schlegel, J.V., Pipkin, G.E., Nishimura, R. & Schultz, G.N. (1970): *J. Urol.* **103**, 155.
Schrauzer, G.N. & Rhead, W.J. (1973): *Int. J. Vit. Res.* **43**, 201.
Smith, L.H. (1972): *New Engl. J. Med.* **287**, 412.
Sorensen, D.I., Devine, M.M. & Rivers, J.M. (1974): *J. Nutr.* **104**, 1041.
Spector, R. (1977): *New Engl. J. Med.* **296**, 1393.
Stich, H.F., Karim, J., Koropatnick, J. & Lo, L. (1976): *Nature, Lond.* **260**, 722.
Stone, I. (1965): *Am. J. Phys. Anthropol.* **23**, 83.
Stone, I. (1966*a*): *Acta Gen. Med. et Gemell.* **15**, 52.
Stone, I. (1966*b*): *Persp. Bio. Med.* **10**, 133.
Stone, I. (1967): *Acta Gen. Med. Gemell.* **16**, 52.
Street, J.C. & Chadwick, R.W. (1975): *Ann. N.Y. Acad. Sci.* **258**, 132.
Subramanian, N. (1977): *Life Sciences* **20**, 1479.
Tas. S. (1976): *Exp. Gerontol.* **11**, 17.
Tatum, J.H., Shaw, P.E. & Berry, R.E. (1969): *J. Agric. Fd Chem.* **17**, 38.
Taylor, G.F. (1968): In *Vitamins in the elderly,* ed A.N. Exton-Smith & D.L. Scott, p. 51. Bristol: John Wright.
Thewlis, B.H. (1974): In *Vitamin C,* ed G.G. Birch & K. Parker, p. 150. London: Applied Science Publishers.
Turley, S.D., West, C.E. & Horton, B.J. (1976): *Atherosclerosis* **24**, 1.
Tyrrell, D.A.J. (1974): *Prescribers' Journal* **14**, 21.
van Eekelen, M. (1936): *Biochem. J.* **30**, 2291.
Vestal, R.E., Norris, A.H., Tobin, J.D., Cohen, B.H., Shock, N.W. & Andres, R. (1975): *Clin. Pharmacol. Ther.* **18**, 425.
Weisburger, J.H. (1977): *Lancet* **2**, 607.
Williams, R.J. & Deason, G. (1967): *Proc. Nat. Acad. Sci.* **57**, 1638.
Williams, Rh. S. & Hughes, R.E. (1972): *Br. J. Nutr.* **28**, 167.
Wilson, C.W.M. (1974): In *Vitamin C,* ed G.G. Birch & K. Parker, p. 203. London: Applied Science Publishers.
Wilson, T.S. (1973): *Age Ageing* **2**, 163.
Wolff, I.A. & Wasserman, A.E. (1972): *Science* **177**, 15.
Wyngaarden, J.B. & Elder, T.D. (1966): In *The metabolic basis of inherited disease,* 2nd edn, ed J.B. Stanbury, J.B. Wyngaarden & D.S. Fredrickson, p. 189. New York: McGraw-Hill.

Yew, M.L.S. (1975): *Ann. N.Y. Acad. Sci.*258, 451.
Zannoni, V.G., Flynn, E.J. & Lynch, M.M. (1972): *Biochem. Pharmacol.* 21, 1377.
Zannoni, V.G. & Sato, P.H. (1976): *Fed. Proc.* 35, 2464.
Zannoni, V.G., Sato, P.H. & Rikans, L.E. (1978): In *Nutrition and drug interrelations,* ed J.N. Hathcock & J. Coon, p. 347. New York: Academic Press.

4

Nutritional aspects of calcium and vitamin D

B.E.C. Nordin.

Introduction

The record of evolution is largely contained in the mineralised tissues, the development of which can be traced back about 500 million years. These mineralised tissues, which include bone, shells and teeth, are generally composed of, or contain, calcium carbonate or calcium phosphate, the latter being the principal mineral constituent of the vertebrate skeleton that we know today and which provides the rigid framework of the human body. Bone comprises about 60 per cent calcium phosphate and 40 per cent collagen and other soft tissues, including cells, and constitutes a remarkable tissue which is almost as strong as cast iron but very much lighter and more elastic (Bell, 1969-70).

Bone is a living tissue which takes part in many of the metabolic processes of the body. It may be secondarily affected by systemic diseases, such as infections, or may develop primary disorders of its own. In either case, skeletal remains provide a fascinating and vital record of the diseases of antiquity and tell us that arthritis, syphilis and many other diseases have affected mankind for a very long time. In particular, it seems that the two main types of primary bone disease we know today – rickets/osteomalacia and osteoporosis – have occurred for many millennia, and it has even been suggested (Ivanhoe, 1970) that some of the physical features of Neanderthal man may be attributable to rickets.

Rickets is a disorder in which, owing to low plasma calcium and/or phosphorus levels, new bone and cartilage fail adequately to mineralise, and deformities of the bones gradually develop. It is generally due to a vitamin D deficiency – though there are rarer forms from other causes – and affects infants and young children during their growing phase. The corresponding condition in the adult is known as osteomalacia. Osteoporosis, on the other hand, represents a reduction in the amount of bone present in the skeleton without any known change in its chemical composition. The bones are therefore more porous than normal although their external dimensions are unchanged. This condition can be produced experimentally in animals by calcium deficiency (Nordin, 1960) and it is probable that the human disease which is a common feature of ageing is also due to negative calcium balance (Nordin, 1961) though not to simple dietary deficiency of calcium (Nordin, 1971).

Rickets

It seems that rickets did not occur during the Egyptian civilisation, though there are references to it in the records of the Roman Empire (Bourke, 1971). Its modern history dates from the 17th century when it was well described by Glisson (1650) in this country, and it became extremely common during the late 19th and early 20th centuries. In the UK it occurred particularly in urban areas (Loomis, 1967) and was frequently referred to on the Continent as 'the English disease' although it was also very prevalent in the USA (Hess, 1930) and in Germany, where most children coming to post-mortem showed some evidence of rickets (Schmorl, 1909).

The association between rickets and urban conditions was long ago shown to be attributable to lack of sunlight. It was found that the incidence was particularly high in cities like Glasgow where the hours of sunlight were among the shortest of any city in the world. It was soon established that rickets could be cured by exposing children or experimental animals to sunlight, and that this could be reproduced by exposure to ultra-violet radiation at 280-310 mμ. It was subsequently established that only 1.5 minutes of such irradiation was required to cure experimental rickets in white rats, and that a longer period was required to achieve the same effect in black rats (Hess, 1930).

The beneficial effects of irradiation are now known to be due to the activation of 7-dehydrocholesterol to cholecalciferol, which occurs in the skin or may be produced *in vitro* by irradiating the precursor in milk or other foodstuffs. More recently, it has been established that even cholecalciferol is not the active form of vitamin D, and that there are further metabolites – 25-hydroxycholecalciferol (produced in the liver) and 1,25-dihydroxycholecalciferol (produced in the kidney) (de Luca, 1969; Fraser & Kodicek, 1970; Gray, Boyle & de Luca, 1971).

The activation of vitamin D precursors in the skin represents an important, if not the major, source of vitamin D for man and it seems likely that more energy is required to produce this effect in pigmented than in fair skins. Loomis (1967) has suggested that the pale skin of the Europeans and Scandinavians represents an adaptation to an environment in which the effective solar irradiation is much less than that to which the original dark skinned humans, who originated nearer the Equator, were accustomed. In fact, osteomalacia due to malabsorption of vitamin D can be treated with ultra-violet irradiation which produces a rapid response of the plasma calcium and phosphorus levels and of the Ca x P product as shown in Fig. 1. The curative effect of a one-month course of artificial sunlight lasts about six months. In view of the critical importance of solar irradiation, the relative scarcity of vitamin D in our diet (see below) and the relatively short hours of sunlight in the United Kingdom, it is perhaps regrettable that Vitaglass, specially manufactured to transmit the ultra-violet radiation which

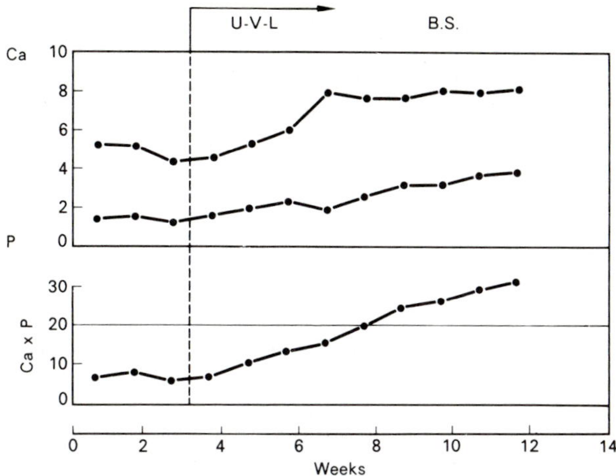

Fig. 1. The effect of a course of artificial sunlight on the mean plasma calcium, phosphate and Ca x P product in a case of osteomalacia with steatorrhoea

is absorbed by ordinary glass, is no longer produced; it was discontinued during the war and has never been resumed.

Rickets is no longer a major problem in this country (except among Asian immigrants) largely due to the fortification of baby foods and dried milk with vitamin D since 1945, the dramatic effect of which is shown in Fig. 2. The vitamin D was originally added to the milk powder in a concentration of 280 units per ounce but a severe epidemic of infantile hypercalcaemia (Lightwood, 1952) – indistinguishable from vitamin D poisoning – necessitated the reduction of this to 115 units per ounce in 1957 (British Paediatric Association, 1956) since when this disease has virtually disappeared. This has been followed by some recrudescence of rickets in Glasgow and other cities (Arneil & Crosbie, 1963) particularly among the immigrant population, but nutritional rickets is still a relatively uncommon disease in this country.*

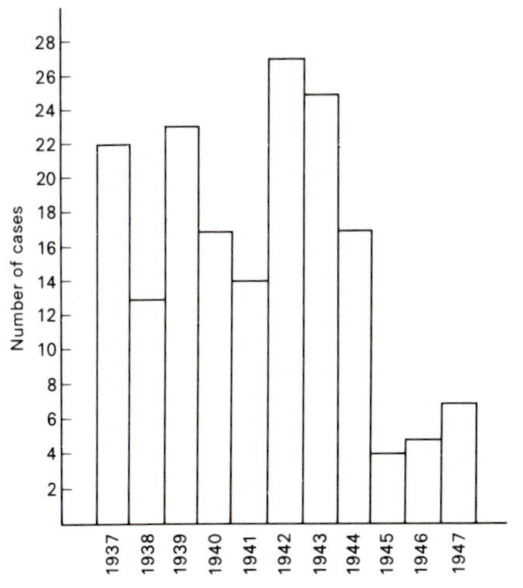

Fig. 2. Annual admissions for rickets to a unit at the Hospital for Sick Children, Glasgow, showing the effect of fortification of baby foods with vitamin D in 1945 (data supplied by G.C. Arneil)

See p. 134 (paragraph c)

Milk and growth

There is no evidence of vitamin D deficiency among white school children in this country, but the obvious need for calcium during growth calls for a consideration of the adequacy of calcium intakes at this time of life.

The average calcium intake in the UK rose from about 600 mg per head per day in 1909 to about 1150 mg in 1960 (Greaves & Hollingsworth, 1966). At the same time, the protein intake has changed very little, perhaps from 75 to 80 g, and the energy intake likewise has only risen by about 10 per cent. During this period, the average height of 12-year-old urban schoolboys has risen by about 2 inches (Boyne, 1960; Tanner, Whitehouse & Takaishi, 1966) (Fig. 3). It is

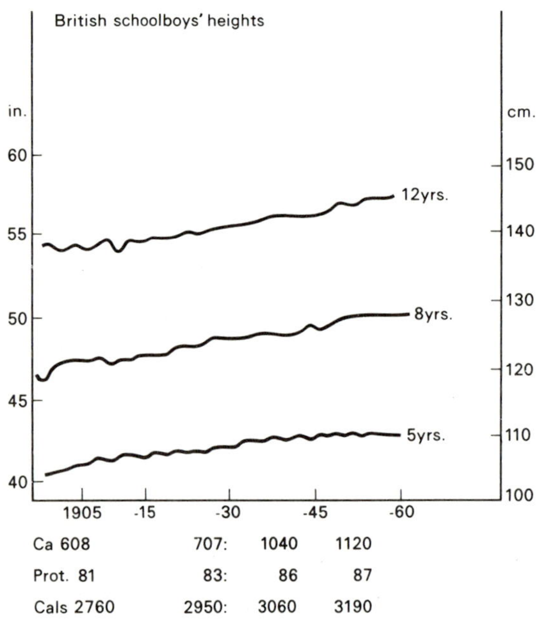

Fig. 3. The mean heights of British schoolboys from 1900 to 1960 together with the estimated calcium, protein and energy intakes over the same period
(Ca = mg/d, Prot. = g/d)

generally thought that this accelerated growth is attributable to the general improvement in nutrition, particularly to energy and protein intake, but it is noteworthy that the proportionate increase in calcium intake has been very much greater than that in protein and energy and this does suggest the possibility that calcium may be playing a significant part in growth. The importance of supplementary milk was in fact demonstrated by Leighton & McKinlay (1930) when they reported on a large scale trial in Lanarkshire in which 10 000 schoolchildren were given extra milk daily for four months and their heights compared with those of 10 000 controls. In all age groups, the milk supplemented children grew significantly faster in the 4-month period than the controls (Fig. 4). It is of course true that the milk will have provided other additional nutrients besides calcium, particularly riboflavin, but the addition of milk to any normal diet produces a very much greater proportionate increase in calcium intake than in that of other nutrients. Milk normally contributes about 47 per cent of the calcium to the national diet but only about 18 per cent of the protein and 10 per cent of the energy (National Food Survey, 1969). It is interesting in this

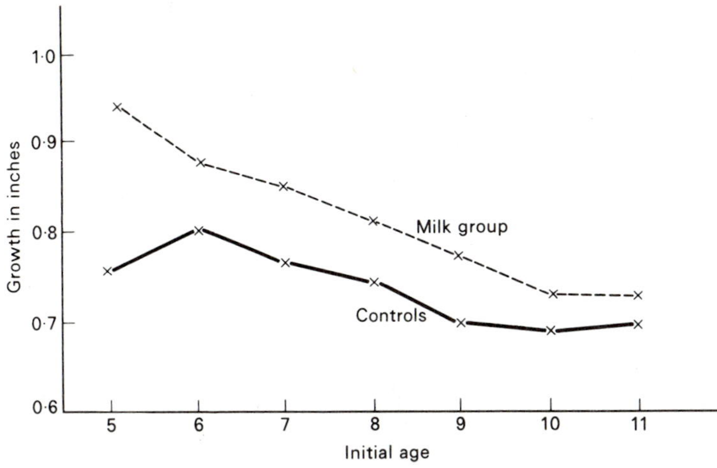

Fig. 4. The effect of ¾ pint of milk, daily for four months, on growth of Lanark schoolchildren (Leighton & McKinlay, 1930)

connection that a recent Indian report suggests improved growth in children given extra calcium (Rajalakshmi, Merchant & Gandhi, 1977).

Certain Japanese data lend further support to the concept that milk, and particularly calcium, may be an important factor in growth. Until about 1950, the calcium intake of the Japanese people was about the lowest in the world – 200 mg per head (Japanese Ministry of Health, 1962), whereas the protein intake was about 60 g and total energy intake about 2000 kcal (8.4 MJ). At about this time the Japanese authorities took steps to remedy this and arrangements were made to fortify school bread and issue free milk to schoolchildren. At the same time, efforts were made to increase milk production and consumption in Japan with the result that calcium intake has risen three-fold in the last 20 years, whereas protein and energy intakes have risen very little. These developments have been associated with an astonishing increase in the mean height of Japanese school-children, 12-year-old boys being now about 4 inches taller than boys of the same age 20 years ago (Japan Statistical Year Book, 1970). Taken in conjunction with the common observation that the children of Japanese immigrants in the United States are usually substantially taller than their parents, this suggests that the small stature of the Japanese is not wholly or even principally due to genetic factors but is probably nutritional in origin, and points to milk, and in particular calcium, as being the relevant nutrient.

These data are relevant to the discontinuance in the UK of infant welfare milk and free school milk for children over seven. Since milk contributes about 47 per cent of the dietary calcium, and since the welfare and school milk comprise about 47 per cent of the total milk intake of the average three-children family (National Health Survey, 1969), it appears that the calcium intake of the average school child may have fallen from 930 to 750 mg unless the parents make up the milk at their own expense or the children to take in additional calcium from other foods. It seems that there is no increase in milk sales during school holidays, which suggests that parents normally do not make up for the milk not provided at school (National Food Survey, Monthly Digest of Statistics, HMSO).

Even more important may be the reported fact that a large proportion of all children who take milk rely on school milk for their only source of this nourishment (Lynch & de la Paz, 1971). If this is correct, it would seem that although the average child is unlikely to suffer any ill effects from the abolition of welfare and school milk, children whose intakes are at the lower end of the normal distribution, and perhaps rely on school milk for most of their dietary calcium, might be reduced to a calcium intake level which could affect growth. However, the Department of Health and Social Security is monitoring a sample of children to detect any effect that may arise.

Calcium in young adults

During adult life, the calcium intake should be sufficient to preserve calcium balance and to maintain an intact skeleton. The amount of calcium required to do this has been repeatedly estimated from balance procedures and found to be about 10/mg/kg, or about 500 mg, per day (Fig. 5). This is an average value,

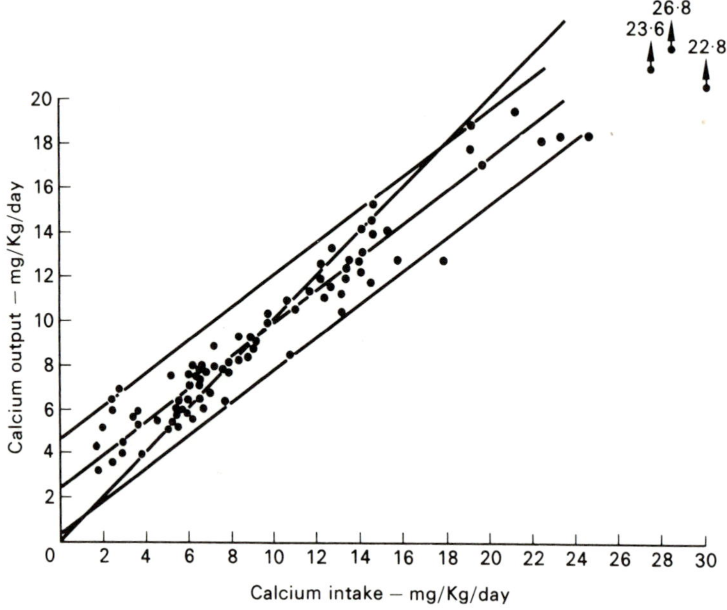

Fig. 5. The relation between calcium intake and calcium output in 92 balances on 39 normal subjects showing that the mean value at which intake and output are equal is about 10 mg/kg

meaning that 50 per cent of adults fall below and 50 per cent above this figure. It is possible that normal people can 'adapt' to lower intakes than this, but the most reliable study on this subject showed that the average requirement even of fully 'adapted' young men was about 420 mg (Malm, 1958). Moreover, such adaptation involves a varying period of negative calcium balance and it is impossible to say what the skeleton may suffer during this period, or whether bone that has been lost can be replaced. It therefore seems unwise to base calcium allowances on the requirement of fully adapted young men and probably wise to adopt the more usual figure of about 500 mg. This is, however, a *requirement* and not an *allowance** (Whedon, 1964). That is to say if all young adults consumed 500 mg calcium a day half of them would in theory be in positive and half in negative balance. From a knowledge of the statistical distribution of calcium requirement and the distribution of dietary intake (both of which have a coefficient of variation of about 25 per cent) it is possible to estimate that the calcium allowance which would protect 95 per cent of the normal population would have to be at least 1 g (Marshall, Nordin & Speed, 1976). This compares with the 500 mg calcium allowance recommended by the British Panel on Recommended Allowances of Nutrients (Department of Health and Social Security, 1969)†, which in turn seems to have been largely based upon the recommendations of the FAO/WHO panel (Food and Agricultural Organisation, 1962). Neither of these committees quoted the published work on calcium requirement and both seem to rely largely upon the assumption that the low calcium intakes in many parts of the world are not associated with any ill effects. As has already been indicated, however, the low calcium intake in Japan may well have been associated with impaired growth and possibly also with a high incidence of osteoporosis (Nordin, 1964).

It is particularly interesting to note how markedly calcium differs from other mineral nutrients in regard to its relatively high requirement. The body responds to deprivation of other minerals by reducing urinary excretion, either through a reduction in plasma concentration or by increasing tubular reabsorption – or both. The result is that very low intakes are required to produce negative sodium, potassium, magnesium or phosphorus balance. Calcium is different from these elements in two respects. First, it is relatively poorly absorbed and at low intakes the faecal calcium actually exceeds the dietary calcium. Secondly, the homeostatic mechanisms prevent a fall in plasma calcium in order to protect the neuromuscular system. Because the plasma calcium cannot fall, calcium continues to be excreted in the urine, the mean minimum value being about 100 - 150 mg/day. This combination of incomplete absorption with obligatory excretion produces the relatively high *mean* requirement of about 500 mg (Marshall *et al.*, 1976).

Calcium stone disease

One of the difficulties in trying to establish the optimum calcium intake of young adults is the clear evidence of an association between calcium stone disease and a high rate of calcium excretion in the urine (Flocks, 1939; Bulusu *et al.*, 1970) which is sometimes taken to mean that the calcium intake in our society is too high. The modern disease of calcium stones in the kidney is not the same as the stone disease of Antiquity and the Middle Ages which was predominantly a bladder stone containing a high proportion of urate (Lonsdale, Sutor & Wooley, 1968). This bladder stone disease has largely disappeared from Western countries as the nutritional status has risen, but it remains a problem in Thailand, the Sudan and other poorer countries and is not yet fully understood (Andersen, 1969).

Calcium stone disease of the kidney now affects about 1-2 per cent of the population at some time in their lives and is particularly prevalent in young adult men. About 50 per cent of these cases have hypercalciuria which is generally due

**See chapter 11* †*The 1979 DHSS recommendations are unchanged except for 1 to 8-year-olds (up from 500 to 600 mg)*

to high absorption of calcium rather than to a high calcium intake (Peacock & Nordin, 1969). This high urine calcium renders them more liable to precipitate calcium oxalate and/or calcium phosphate in the urine as the result of over-saturation (Fig. 6). Moreover, the urine oxalate tends to be raised as well.

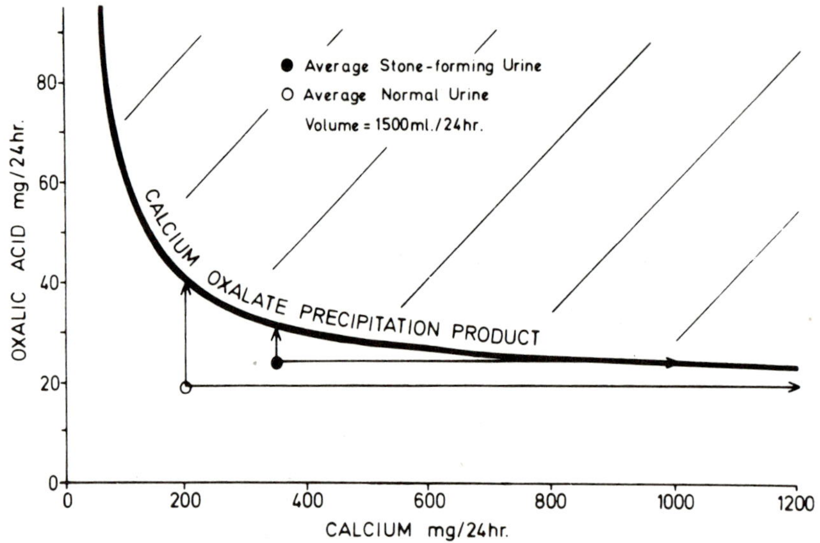

Fig. 6. The relation between calcium and oxalate output in average stone-forming and average normal urine to indicate how much nearer the stone-former is to the calcium oxalate product at which precipitation will occur. The figure also shows that a rise in urine oxalate is more liable to produce precipitation than a rise in urine calcium

Although this is not the complete explanation of calcium stone disease, it can be confidently stated that without initial precipitation calcium stones cannot develop, and that precipitation cannot occur from an under-saturated urine. Since it is known that the urinary calcium of such patients can be easily reduced by restricting the calcium intake (Peacock & Nordin, 1969) it seems logical to treat these cases with a low-calcium diet. The results obtained so far in a group of recurrent stone formers observed for up to ten years are shown in the Table below. However, because calcium restriction allows more oxalate to be absorbed and excreted (Nordin *et al.*, 1971) we restrict the oxalate intake as well. The effects of this diet is shown in the Table; clearly it is very effective. Even more impressive is treatment with phosphate supplements which lower urine calcium and increase inhibitory activity in the urine.

It should be added that this dietary restriction should only be applied to

Effect of low-calcium, low-oxalate diet and P supplement on renal stone formation

	Pre-diet	Diet	P supps
Episodes	144	125	20
Patient-years	184	322	79
Episodes/year	0.78	0.38	0.25

young adults with a high calcium absorption and should not be more severe than is required to bring the urinary calcium into the normal range. Over-severe restriction could well lead to negative calcium balance and the regime should probably not be applied to post-menopausal women or other cases in which there is a high obligatory loss of calcium from bone resorption.

The existence of this small, but nonetheless significant, population of hyper-absorbing calcium-stone formers further complicates the question of the recommended calcium intake of young adults. Intakes that may be appropriate for the majority of the population may well be excessive for those with hyper-absorption. Perhaps when preventive medicine is more widely practised, screening procedures will include the measurement of urinary calcium or calcium absorption so that individuals may be given advice on their recommended calcium intake before they have actually developed stone disease. More and more of the risk factors have now been identified, and they include a raised urine calcium, oxalate, pH and uric acid and a lowered excretion of inhibitors. Most of these factors are adversely affected by raising protein intake, and there is a striking world-wide relationship between protein intake and the prevalence of calcium stone disease (Roberston *et al.*, 1978).

Post-menopausal osteoporosis

Loss of bone in women commences soon after the menopause and continues to the end of life at a rate of about 0.5-1.0 per cent of the skeleton per annum, representing a negative calcium balance of about 15-30 mg per day (Nordin, 1971) (Fig. 7). This loss of bone is associated with a startling increase in the lower forearm fracture rate which rises from about five cases per 10 000 per annum in women in the fourth decade to about 50 cases per 10 000 in the seventh decade. There is no corresponding increase in the forearm fracture rate in men (Knowelden, Buhr & Dunbar, 1964).

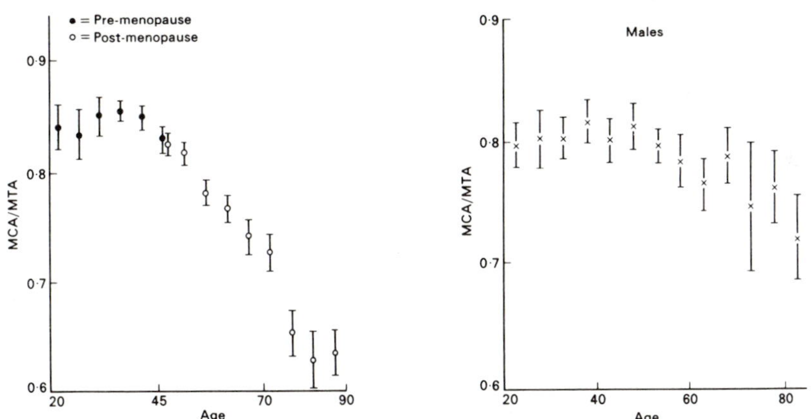

Fig. 7. Metacarpal cortical area/total area ratios as a function of age: in normal women (left) and normal men (right)

This loss of bone is due to an increase in bone resorption which, however, is generally too small to cause a detectable rise in the 24-hour urine calcium, which is largely derived from absorbed dietary calcium. However, the rise in calcium excretion is apparent in the early morning fasting urine and is associated with a small increase in plasma calcium, both of which features can be clearly seen after an artificial menopause (Gallagher, Young & Nordin, 1972). These biochemical manifestations of increased bone resorption can be reversed by replacement therapy with oestrogenic hormones and such therapy prevents post-menopausal bone loss (Aitken *et al.*, 1973) which can also be substantially delayed by administration of calcium supplements (Horsman *et al.*, 1977; Recker, Saville & Heaney, 1977). A recent study shows that such treatment reduces fracture rates in post-menopausal women (Hutchison, Polansky & Feinstein, 1979).

The reason for the post-menopausal increase in bone resorption seems to be that bone becomes more sensitive to parathyroid hormone in the absence of oestrogens. The parathyroid glands secrete this hormone in response to a falling or reduced plasma calcium, which normally maintains the concentration at about 10 mg/100 ml by increasing calcium absorption, decreasing calcium excretion – and if necessary – increasing bone resorption. During the daytime, and on a normal diet, significant bone resorption is probably not required to maintain the plasma calcium, but since the absorption of calcium appears to be completed within about six hours of the average meal (Birge *et al.*, 1969) it is probable that such bone resorption is required to maintain the plasma calcium between about midnight and breakfast time. In pre-menopausal women, the bone is relatively insensitive to parathyroid hormone which exerts its maximum effect upon tubular resorption of calcium in the kidney, thus reducing calcium excretion to a minimum before resorbing bone (Nordin & Peacock, 1969). In post-menopausal women, the increased sensitivity of bone to parathyroid hormone (and probably also to $1{,}25(OH)_2 D_3$) causes more calcium to be resorbed from bone and excreted in the urine. Hence the slightly raised fasting plasma and urinary calcium of post-menopausal women.

These observations and this hypothesis raise the question of whether replacement therapy with small doses of oestrogens should be more common during the post-menopausal period. Such therapy is widely practised in the United States and on the Continent, but in the United Kingdom is less popular though its use is growing. Oestrogens may produce a beneficial effect on general well-being, and improve the epithelium and lubrication of the vagina. Against these advantages must be set the possible hazards, particularly that of thrombosis which has been demonstrated with the large doses of oestrogens used at one time in the contraceptive pill (Inman *et al.*, 1970). There has also been much controversy over reports from the USA of an increased risk of endometrial cancer in patients on oestrogen (Smith *et al.*, 1975). This has not been confirmed by European workers in the field who regard the reports with some reserve. In any event, there is little evidence of such dangers at a dosage of 25 μg daily of ethinyl oestradiol, and it is probable that bone resorption can be adequately controlled at even lower doses at which the risk of side effects must be very small indeed. It should be emphasised that oestrogen therapy must be given on a cyclical basis (for three weeks out of four) to prevent hyperplasia of the endometrium and break-through bleeding.

Since the degree of oestrogen insufficiency varies greatly among post-menopausal women, it would seem logical for the medical profession to look more carefully at oestrogen status and prescribe oestrogens at least in those post-menopausal women in whom there is evidence of genuine deficiency. It is doubtful whether such treatment affects 'ageing', but probable that it could prevent or delay some at least of the degenerative processes which follow the menopause.

Femoral neck fractures
The loss of bone which starts in women at the menopause, and rather later in men, finally reaches the stage at which it causes fractures of the neck of the femur. This reaches a level of some 2 per cent of the female and 1 per cent of the male population per annum in the ninth decade (Knowelden *et al.*, 1964).

This continuing loss of bone is associated with a steady decline in calcium absorption (Bullamore *et al.*, 1970) (Fig. 8) which reflects – in part at least – a

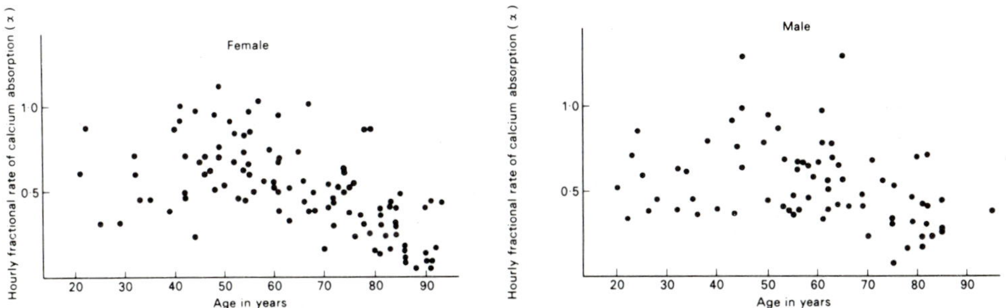

Fig. 8. Radio-calcium absorption as a function of age in: normal women (left) and normal men (right)

fall in plasma 25-OHD_3 levels with age (Fig. 9). Moreover, femoral-neck-fracture cases have even lower plasma 25-OHD_3 levels than other elderly subjects (Fig. 9). The ultimate expression of this vitamin D deficiency is osteomalacia which is surprisingly common among the elderly in the U.K. (Chalmers *et al.*, 1967) and even more common in cases of fractured neck of femur (Aaron *et al.*, 1977). It has already been pointed out that the supply of vitamin D from diet and sunshine is low in this country. Rickets has been abolished by fortifying baby foods with vitamin D, but no corresponding preventive measure has been provided for adults apart from fortification of margarine. Very few other foods, except fatty fish, contain significant amounts of this nutrient. Taken in conjunction with the low plasma vitamin D levels reported in this country by Lumb, Mawer & Stanbury (1971) it seems probable that old people are moving into a state of significant vitamin D deficiency. On the other hand, it is also possible that vitamin D requirement rises with age, either due to general impairment of absorptive function or to declining renal function with impaired conversion of vitamin D to its active metabolite (Fraser & Kodicek, 1970). This could explain why rather large doses of vitamin D seem to be required to reverse malabsorption of calcium in old people.

This does not mean that the whole of the bone loss and increased fracture risk

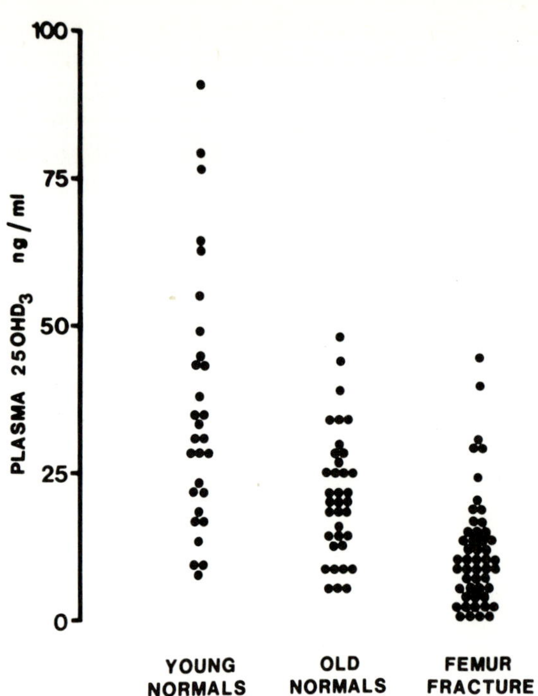

Fig. 9. Plasma 25-OHD$_3$ levels in normal young subjects, normal elderly subjects and cases of femoral neck fracture

of old people can necessarily be attributed to vitamin D deficiency, but even the fracture cases who only have osteoporosis suffer from malabsorption of calcium and it can be argued that this represents a milder form of vitamin D deficiency than is present in the fully developed osteomalacia cases. This milder degree of

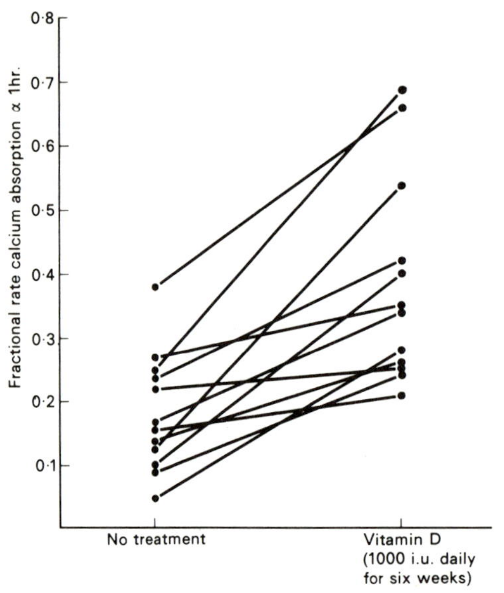

Fig. 10. Effect of vitamin D 1000 units for six weeks on radio-calcium absorption in normal elderly subjects

vitamin D deficiency may produce or aggravate loss of bone by its adverse effect on calcium absorption. This, however, is speculative. The role of vitamin D deficiency in osteomalacia is well established; its role in osteoporosis hypothetical. However, it is a fact that malabsorption of calcium in elderly subjects can be at least partially corrected by quite small doses of vitamin D (Fig. 10) and it is therefore possible that loss of bone in the elderly might be delayed by vitamin D administration.

References

Aaron, J.E., Gallagher, J.C., Anderson, J., Stasiak, L., Longton, E.B., Nordin, B.E.C. & Nicholson, M. (1974): *Lancet* 1, 229.

Aitken, J.M., Hart, D.M. & Lindsay, R. (1973): *Br. Med. J.* 3, 515.

Andersen, D.A. (1969): *Proceedings of renal stone research symposium,* Leeds 1968, ed A. Hodgkinson and B.E.C. Nordin, p. 17. London: Churchill.

Arneil, G.C. & Crosbie, J.C. (1963): *Lancet* 2, 423.

Bell, G.H. (1969-70): *Advancement of Science* 26, 1.

Birge, S.J., Peck, W.A., Berman, M. & Whedon, G.D. (1969): *J. Clin. Invest.* 48, 1705.

Bourke, J.B. (1971): *Med. Hist.* 15, 363.

Boyne, A.W. (1960): *Human growth, III,* ed J.M. Tanner, Oxford: Pergamon Press.

British Paediatric Association (1956): *Br. Med. J.* 2, 149.

Bullamore, J.R., Gallagher, J.C., Wilkinson, R., Nordin, B.E.C. & Marshall, D.H. (1970): *Lancet* 2, 535.

Bulusu, L., Hodgkinson, A., Nordin, B.E.C. & Peacock, M. (1970): *Clin. Sci.* 38, 601.

Chalmers, J., Conachier, W.D.H., Gardner, D.L. & Scott, P.J. (1967): *J. Bone Jt Surg.* **49B**, 403.

DeLuca, H.F. (1969): *Fed. Proc.* 28, 1678.

Department of Health and Social Security (1969): *Recommended intakes of nutrients for the United Kingdom.* Rep. Publ. Hlth Med. Subj. No. 120. London: HMSO.

Flocks, R.H. (1939): *J. Am. Med. Ass.* 113, 1466.

Food and Agriculture Organisation of the United Nations (1962): *Calcium requirements.* FAO Nutrition Meetings Report Series No. 30. Rome.

Fraser, D.R. & Kodicek, E. (1970): *Nature* 228, 764.

Gallagher, J.C., Young, M.M. & Nordin, B.E.C. (1972): *Clin. Endocrinol.* 1, 57.

Glisson, F. (1650): *De rachitide sive morbo puerili, qui vulgo 'The Rickets' Dicitur.* London.

Gray, R., Boyle, I. & DeLuca, H.F. (1971): *Science* 172, 1232.

Greaves, J.P. & Hollingsworth, Dorothy F. (1966): *Wld Rev. Nutr. Dietet.* 6, 34.

Hess, A.F. (1930): *Rickets including osteomalacia and tetany.* London: Henry Kimpton.

Horsman, A., Gallagher, J.C., Simpson, M. & Nordin, B.E.C. (1977): *Br. Med. J.* 2, 789.

Hutchinson, T.A., Polansky, S.M. & Feinstein, A.R. (1979): *Lancet* 2, 705.

Inman, W.H.W., Vessey, M.P., Westerholm, Barbro & Engelun, A. (1970): *Br. Med. J.* 2, 203.

Ivanhoe, F. (1970): *Nature* 227, 577.

Japan Statistical Year Book (1970): Bureau of Statistics Office of the Prime Minister, Tokyo.

Japanese Ministry of Health and Welfare (1962): *Nutrition in Japan.* Tokyo.

Knowelden, J., Buhr, A.J. & Dunbar, Olive (1964): *Br. J. Prev. Soc. Med.* 18, 130.

Leighton, G. & McKinlay, P.L. (1930): *Milk consumption and the growth of school children.* Department of Health for Scotland. London: HMSO.

Lightwood, R. (1952): *Archs Dis. Childh.* 27, 302.

Lonsdale, K., Sutor, J. & Wooley, S. (1968): *Br. J. Urol.* 40, 33.

Loomis, W.F. (1967): *Science* 157, 501.

Lumb, G.A., Mawer, E.B. & Stanbury, S.W. (1971): *Am. J. Med.* 50, 421.

Lynch, G. & de la Paz, Sylvia (1971): *New Scientist* 51, (758), 32.

Malm, O.J. (1958): *Scand. J. Clin. Lab. Invest.* 10, Suppl. 36.

Marshall, D.H., Nordin, B.E.C. & Speed, R. (1976): *Proc. Nutr. Soc.* 35, 163.

Ministry of Agriculture, Fisheries and Food (1969): *Household food consumption and expenditure, 1967.* Annual report of the National Food Survey Committee. London: HMSO.

Ministry of Agriculture, Fisheries and Food. *National Food Survey. Monthly Digest of Statistics.* London: HMSO.

Nordin, B.E.C. (1960): *Clin. Orthopaed.* **17**, 235.

Nordin, B.E.C. (1961): *Lancet* **1**, 1011.

Nordin, B.E.C. (1964): *The relation between dietary calcium and osteoporosis in different parts of the world.* Report to the Nutrition Section of the World Health Organisation.

Nordin, B.E.C. (1971): *Br. Med. J.* **1**, 571.

Nordin, B.E.C., Hodgkinson, A., Peacock, M. & Robertson, W.G. (1971): The medical treatment of renal stone disease. In *Xe Congres International de Therapeutique,* p. 191. Paris: Doin.

Nordin, B.E.C. & Peacock, M. (1969): *Lancet* **2**, 1280.

Peacock, M. & Nordin, B.E.C. (1969): The hypercalciuria of renal stone disease. In *Proceedings of renal stone research symposium, Leeds 1968.* ed A. Hodgkinson and B.E.C. Nordin. London: Churchill.

Rajalakshmi, R., Merchant, G.V. & Gandhi, V.H. (1977): *Baroda J. Nutr.* **4**, 51.

Recker, R.R., Saville, P.D. & Heaney, R.P. (1977): *Ann. Inter. Med.* **87**, 649.

Roberston, W.G., Peacock, M., Heyburn, P., Speed, R. & Hanes, F. (1978): *Fortschr. Urol. Nephrol.* **11**, 5.

Schmorl, G. (1909): *Ergebn. Inn. Med. Kinderheilk.* **4**, 403.

Smith, D.C., Prentice, R., Thompson, D.J. & Herrman, W.L. (1975): *New Engl. J. Med.* **293**, 1164.

Tanner, J.M., Whitehouse, R.H. & Takaishi, M. (1966): *Archs Dis. Childh.* **41**, 454.

Whedon, G.D. (1964): The combined use of balance and isotopic studies in the study of calcium metabolism. In *Proceedings of the Sixth International Congress of Nutrition, 1963.* p.425. Edinburgh: Livingstone.

5

Dietary fibre

M. A. Eastwood.

Introduction : historical aspects

Dietary fibre is enjoying a renaissance in human nutrition (Anon, 1977), but as the interest in the subject grows so does the confusion. This is because of the complexity of the subject.

The development of nutrition as a science owes much to the isolation and characterisation of individual substances of nutritional importance. Their absorption was found to take place in the upper small intestine. For such absorption to take place it is necessary for there to be a systematic enzymatic breakdown of the complex foods in the gut to simple entities, eg amino acids, sugars and fatty acids. The recognition of this process enabled an understanding of digestion, which in turn lead to improved nutrition. As a result of this the assumption grew that molecules of large molecular weight had to be broken down in the intestine, and subsequently absorbed, in order to be nutritionally significant. Substances of large molecular weight, eg protein, were readily evaluated in terms of their amino-acid constituents.

Complex polysaccharides and lignins did not appear to be essential or relevant to nutrition as they appeared to resist digestion. Consequently, these substances were increasingly ignored. This loss of interest was given impetus by a changing clinical attitude to fibre. The addage 'an apple a day keeps the doctor away' had been used by clinicians in various circumstances since the beginning of medicine. The value of cereal bran, fruit and vegetables in preventing constipation was recognised in both ancient and mediaeval times.

During this century there has been a profound social change in that the woman of the house works in the kitchen often in addition to an outside job and is enabled to do this by virtue of appliances and convenience foods. These convenience foods have followed the dictates of known nutrition and have been complete in terms of energy intake and essential proteins, vitamins and trace elements and possessing prolonged storage life. Such properties have not suggested the need for complex plant fibres.

In the 1920s and 1930s there wan an attempt by Kellogg in the United States and Allinson in Great Britain to alter the existing trend but which only served to accentuate it. They suggested that a largely vegetarian diet was highly desirable for health. Their approach, along with others, was dismissed as crankish. As a result fibre disappeared from the clinician's regime. Low-residue diets became the vogue in gastroenterology. and the removal of roughage from the diet was the common response to clinical problems, eg diarrhoea. The concept developed of plant fibre passing along the gastrointestinal tract like a wire wool pad excoriating the wall. Only the fit could resist such an insult. If fibre was of any value then it was a useful laxative with devotees taking commercially available cereal bran preparations (Alvarez, 1949).

The ruminant physiologists continued to be aware of the importance of fibre for in order to develop efficient farming it is necessary to adequately feed the stock. The ruminant physiologists described fibre both in chemical and physiological terms and at the same time developed appropriate chemical and physical analytical methods (van Soest & McQueen, 1973).

In man there were a few experiments on fibre and bowel action (Williams & Olmsted, 1936; Hoppert & Clark, 1945). McCance & Widdowson (1955) studied the physiological effect of brown and white bread when passing along the gastrointestinal tract. Malhotra (1968) suggested that fibre might protect against coronary heart disease. Kritchevsky (1964), Portman (1960) and Moore (1967) showed that plant fibre could protect against atherogenic diets in experimental animals.

Then Commander Cleave, a retired Naval Medical Officer, linked the development of the diseases that are so much part of our modern clinical experience with the high sucrose, low-fibre content of our diet. His book (Cleave, Campbell & Painter, 1966) attracted the interest of Denis Burkitt (1973) and Hugh Trowell (1973) who had worked for many years in East Africa. The belief of these clinicians was that in Africa such diseases as coronary heart disease, diabetes mellitus, hiatus hernia, appendicitis, cancer of the colon, diverticular disease, constipation, varicose veins and pulmonary embolism were rarely seen. They ascribed the absence of these problems to the high fibre content of the African diet. In contrast the low fibre content of the European and North American diet was an important factor in the aetiology of these diseases. The gastrointestinal diseases were associated with a prolonged gastrointestinal transit time, stasis of gastrointestinal contents of the sigmoid colon and passage of a small faecal stool. This was in contrast with exuberant defaecation habits of the rural African who was free of these diseases. The dietary fibre hypothesis (see Figure) was given a fillip by the observation by Painter (1975) that fibre in the form of bran was of value in the treatment of the symptoms of diverticular disease. This was a reversal of the low-fibre regime. This however was a therapeutic advance rather than a confirmation of aetiological factors.

We are no closer to confirming or disproving this hypothesis than at the outset, but interesting observations have accrued which have considerable clinical and therapeutic import. Furthermore, unexpected areas of ignorance in many branches of nutrition and gastroenterology have been exposed as a result of the questions posed by the studies in fibre. For example, most intestinal absorption studies have been conducted using solutions, whereas in life the substances are

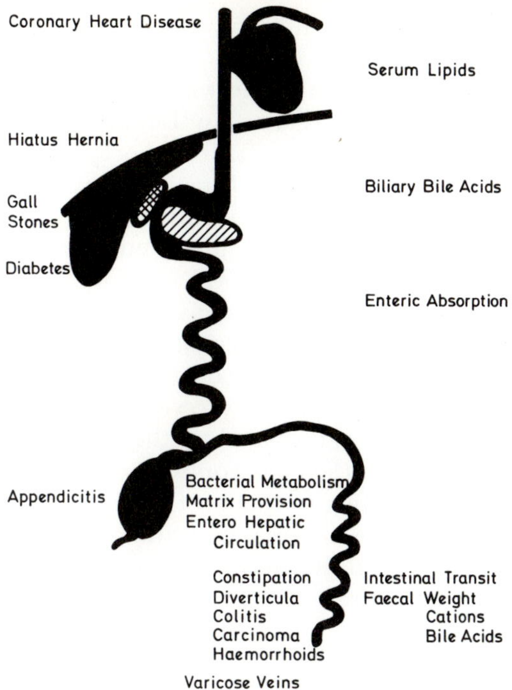

Fig. 1. Dietary fibre hypothesis

absorbed from a viscous mud which constitutes the ingested meal. The rate of absorption from such a complex is unlikely to be the same as from a pure solution.

What is fibre? Trowell (1975) defined fibre as skeletal remains of plant cells that are resistant to digestion by the enzymes of man. He also suggested the term dietary fibre, a name which is easily understood and places no preconceptions in an area involving knowledge.

The understanding of fibre in the diet is bedevilled by the historical problems associated with the measurement of fibre and also by the large variety of cereals, fruit and vegetables eaten by man. The fruit and vegetables that we eat are either roots, stalks, leaves or flowers and it is unlikely that the chemistry of different varieties and the anatomical portions that we eat are uniformly the same.

The climatic conditions under which these plants are grown, the season of the year and the condition of the soil are almost certainly liable to change the chemistry of the fibrous material. The plant at the time it is eaten is a complex structure, with secondary thickening and a varying degree of and lignification of the cell wall. The plant consists of an orderly structure consisting of pith, xylem and phloem, made up of polysaccharides and lignin material. Secondary cell wall is laid in the primary or initial cell wall as a continuous layer or as localised thickening or bands, particularly in the cells of the xylem. A major source of plant fibre is bran which is a by-product of the flour milling process. It consists of the outer layer of the wheat germ and includes the aleurone layer. The bran constitutes between 11 and 16 per cent of the wheat as it is harvested. It consists of the epidermis, cuticle and cross-cell and tube-cell layers, and the seed coat.

The histological and chemical nature of bran will vary considerably depending on the milling conditions (Cummings, 1976).

The early days of the renaissance of interest in fibre were bedevilled by the use of a method of analysing fibre developed by Einhof in 1806, which measure the crude fibre content of animal foodstuffs. It was originally used to detect the adulteration of foodstuffs with sawdust. Unfortunately it has no place as a predictor of the nutritive value of fibre. The use of this term is not to be recommended in any studies of vegetable dietary fibre in human nutrition (Southgate, 1976).

The problems, however, in measuring the constituents of fibre are formidable. Fibre consists of a polymeric mass with the constituent polysaccharides and lignin intermeshed; they can only be separated each from the other by solvents of varying severity. Much of the data relating to vegetable dietary fibre is derived from wood, cereal and grasses and is provided by the ruminant physiologists. There is very little information on the commonly eaten fruit and vegetables. One of the considerable problems relating to dietary fibre is that the method of preparation can considerably alter the material with the possibilities of artefacts developing. There is also the possibility of inadvertent hydrolysis of the polysaccharides by extraction procedure.

Chemical constituents of fibre (Rees, 1967)

Cellulose

Cellulose is a widely distributed polymer. It consists of unbranched, 1-4β glucose polymers consisting of 3000 to 100 000 glucose units resulting in the molecular weight of more than 600 000. The cellulose strands consist of flattened ribbon structures which may cross-link with other substances, but the linear shape is preserved. This means that cellulose forms a three-dimensional lattice work woven into the cell wall. The cellulose is susceptible to cellulases produced by fungi or bacteria but it is believed that mammals are not capable of hydrolysing cellulose.

Hemicelluloses or pentosans

These substances are also known as non-cellulosic polysaccharides. They are characterised by a lack of uniformity in their structure, being complex polymers of hexose sugars which may branch. They have a varying solubility in alkali so that they present considerable problems in analysis. After extraction in weak alkali, adding acid yields hemicellulose A or ethanol hemicellulose B. An alternative classification is acidic and neutral hemicelluloses; some of the hemicelluloses are without acidic sugars. Essentially, the hemicelluloses consist of a backbone xylose sugar with arabinose, mannose, glucose, galactose, rhamnose, galacturonic acid randomly distributed through the polymer. In general the units are between 150-200 sugar units in size. The polymers are readily hydrolysed by weak acid. The neutral hemicelluloses are to be found in cereal fibre and there is a variable xylose-to-arabinose ratio depending on the type of cereal. The acidic hemicelluloses, however, are somewhat smaller in molecular weight but are more highly branched.

Pectin
Pectins are present in much smaller amounts but are common to most cell walls representing 1-4 per cent of the total cell-wall polysaccharides. Except for certain specialist tissues, such as the skin of citrus fruits, it is a somewhat ill-defined group with a molecular weight of 60 000 - 90 000. Pectins are soluble in hot water, but are present in plants usually as the calcium salts, therefore EDTA is used in their extraction to remove the calcium. Pectins are of great interest to industry because of their ability to form gels.

Essentially, pectins are polymerised 1-4β-D-galacturonic acids though they also contain D-galactose and L-aribinose. These neutral sugars may constitute 10-25 per cent of the polymer. The acidic sugars may be methylated to a varying degree which can affect their physiological functions. The pectins may be homo-polysaccharides, containing principally one sugar polymer, or more usually they are heteropolysaccharide pectin which is a much more complex structure.

Plant gums and mucillages
These are storage polysaccharides and whilst they are not strictly cell-wall components they have biochemical and physical properties similar to the plant-wall constituents. Plant gums are exudates which form at the site of injury to plants which try to give a protection to plants. They are used commercially by the food industry as emulsifiers, thickeners and stabilisers. They are a complex group of highly-branched uronic-acid polymers, principally glucuronic and galacturonic acid. Gum arabic is perhaps the best known plant gum. Another plant gum, sterculia, which is obtained from India, is a galacturonic acid polymer but includes D-galactose and L-rhaminose residues. Mucillages are mixed in with the endosperm or storage polysaccharides of plant seeds and retain water. They are present in plants to prevent drying out. These are mostly neutral polysaccharides with occasional acidic groups present. Other storage polysaccharides include inulin which is found in dahlia tubers and the Jerusalem artichoke.

Lignin
Lignin is not a polysaccharide but a phenyl-propane polymer. Links between the basic units are complex. The lignin is probably attached to the polysaccharide. It is present in large amounts in wood where it may constitute 40-50 per cent of the cell wall, whereas in wheat cell walls, cabbage and apple it is found only in trace amounts. Most of our knowledge about the chemistry of lignin is derived from studies on wood. Our knowledge of the chemistry of lignin in commonly eaten fruit and vegetables is sparse.

To an extent, however, the classification of components of the plant cell wall is based on classical schemes of fractionation. Each method used to fractionate the plant cell wall may yield different components. In addition the physical properties of those isolates may well be distinct from those from a different but equally logical procedure. It is important, therefore, that even minor modifications from an accepted technique are defined so that the distinctions can be made obvious to someone who is trying to repeat the work.

The analysis of dietary fibre
This presents many problems to the analyst (Southgate, 1976). The methods

used are derived from two sources. One has been evolved by the ruminant physiologist, aware that a significant fraction of many forages are not digested within the mammalian tract. These forages are digested in the ruminant tract which made it necessary for methods to be developed which were unique to the ruminant physiologist.

Crude fibre

This is a method which uses an air-dried sample of food, extracted to remove lipid and then extracted successively with boiling acid and alkali. The residue is filtered, washed, dried and weighed. It will be appreciated that there will be many errors inherent in such a crude method.

Acid detergent fibre and neutral detergent fibre

Van Soest (Van Soest & McQueen, 1973) examined the use of anionic, cationic and non-ionic detergents in producing a fibre with a low nitrogen content. Van Soest was able to show that by selective extraction one could have a preparation which composed largely of hemicellulose, cellulose and lignin depending on the extraction conditions. The neutral detergent fibre results from the extraction of the plant material with a hot neutral solution of the detergent, sodium lauryl sulphate, resulting in a preparation containing cell-wall constituents. The acid-detergent fibre complex measured consists of cellulose and lignin. It results from the heating of the sample with normal sulphuric acid containing cetyl trimethyl-ammonium bromide, the residue being filtered off and washed in the usual way. These are methods which require a great deal of practice but which are very useful. However, their principal use may still remain in animal physiology rather than in human physiology. The neutral-detergent fibre method also has a disadvantage in that there is some loss of hemicelluloses from the prepared material when this method is used for fruit and vegetables. This shortcoming is less apparent in grasses and cereal fibres.

Measurement of constituents of plant cell walls

These second series of methods have been generated as a result of a wish to correlate the constituents of the plant cell wall with the biological effects. A number of analytical methods have been developed but the one which is most applicable is that of Southgate (1976). As it is the most sophisticated it carries with it great demands on time and expertise. On the other hand it is most likely to yield the highest rewards in advancing our knowledge of this subject. As in most of the methods, the fibre is extracted to remove lipids, dried and then carried through a series of procedures which separate out different fractions. Starch is first removed by enzymatic hydrolysis. Following ethanolic precipitation cellulose and pentose and lignins can be estimated. The supernatant is also analysed for water-soluble non-cellulosic polysaccharides. The hydrolysates are analysed for hexoses, pentoses and uronic acid.

Physical properties of fibre

An alternative or complementary approach to understanding the biological function of fibre is to regard it as a physical agent. The physical characteristics which may be of importance in nutrition are water-holding, cation exchange, adsorption, gel-filtration properties and the production of a matrix by the fibre, ie a sponge-like structure (Eastwood & Mitchell, 1976).

Water-holding capacity

Plant-cell materials swell in water to a coherent structure. Some polysaccharides will swell more than others. However, it is difficult to estimate the water-holding capacity because the method of preparation of the fibrous material can affect it. Similarly, some substances when extracted from the plant fibre will swell in a way that they would be able to if modified or constrained by being involved in a mesh with less hydrophilic substances.

When fibre is exposed to water there is adsorption of water in different forms. Surface water covering the fibre is the first layer, thereafter interstitial water fills up the spaces of the fibrous material until the capacity of the interstitial space is filled. Any water thereafter will be free water so that the fibre has a saturation capacity. This capacity is determined not only by the chemistry and the shape of the macromolecules but also the pH and electrolyte concentration of the surrounding liquid.

The main source of variation in water-holding capacity is the type of plant material. There are, however, problems associated with the method of preparation which can alter the water-holding capacity. The surface area of the fibre is important. This area can be altered by the method of preparation so that exposure to organic solvents and the method of drying are subtle variants. If the capillary structure of the fibre collapses with dehydration it may be irreversible. On the other hand, wet fibre is difficult to characterise in terms of surface properties. The fibre contents of different vegetables vary. The fibre content of cucumber is less than 4 per cent whereas bran is 95 per cent fibrous material. The average water content of fruit and vegetables eaten is about 85-90 per cent, therefore it is necessary to eat a great deal of fruit and vegetables to obtain the same amount of fibrous material as from taking bran.

The water-holding capacity of a plant depends not only on its fibre content but also on the water-holding capacity of the particular fibre (McConnell, Eastwood & Mitchell, 1974). For example, rhubarb is 4 per cent dry weight but the fibre in that dry weight will hold 15 g of water/g fibre. Therefore the potential water holding capacity of that rhubarb is 60 g/100 g of raw rhubarb. Yet 100 g of bran will hold 450 g of water. Therefore, theoretically, 50 g of bran is capable of holding 225 g of water which is functionally equivalent to 100 g of raw carrot, 150 g of apple or 200 g of orange pith. These are the vegetable sources which are of greatest value in altering stool weight. However, these estimates may be modified by bacterial sacharolytic activity in the caecum with consequent loss of the matrix structure in the gel.

Ion-exchange capacity

The acidic sugars of polysaccharides give fibre cation-exchange properties. The adsorption of cation to the uronic-acid groups result in changes in the gelling properties and water-holding capacity. Most vegetable fibres are monofunctional weak cation exchangers, eg pear has a capacity of 0.6 m equiv./g dry fibre and turnip, carrot and cabbage have cation-exchange capacities in excess of 2 m equiv./g. Wheat bran, maize, banana and potato fibre are polyfunctional cation exchangers. There does not appear to be any significant anion-exchange capacity (McConnell *et al.*, 1974).

Adsorption of bile acids to fibre
Fibre binds bile acids and this is of interest because bile acids are an important route by which cholesterol is removed from the body. Theoretically, the greater the loss of bile acids from the enterohepatic circulation the lower the serum cholesterol. Free bile acids, eg deoxycholic acid, which are found in the faeces are most strongly adsorbed to fibre. This contrasts with the weaker adsorption of conjugated bile acids such as are found in the jejunum. The adsorption is pH-dependent, being greatest as an acid pH, and appears to be hydrophobic in nature (Eastwood & Hamilton, 1968; Story & Kritchevsky, 1976).

Surface area, pore size, filtration properties
The properties of fibre along the intestine may be likened to that of the chromatographic material. That is that fibre provides a matrix surrounded by water in different phases into which the solute and bacteria may permeate, according to molecular weight, shape and size. Some solutes and bacteria will be adsorbed to the fibre. The fibre may act as a gel.

This description suggests that different fibres will act in different ways. Each fibre may act in a particular way along the gastrointestinal tract affecting absorption and movement of substances within the gastrointestinal tract, depending on the particular physical properties of that fibre. Each fibre source, however, will have a mixture of properties, one of which may be predominant.

The role for fibre along the gastrointestinal tract
Adding fibre to meals delays the gastric emptying time, fluid leaving the stomach more rapidly than the solid phase (McCance & Widdowson, 1955).

Small intestinal absorption
The addition of pectin and guar gum to the diet in modest amounts, 10 g/day, flattens the blood glucose response to oral glucose. Therefore, gelling agents such as guar and pectin are modifiers of absorption. So much so that high-carbohydrate diets, rich in dietary fibre, can modify the treatment requirements of diabetic men, hitherto receiving sulfonylureas and insulin (Jenkins *et al.*, 1977; Kiehm, Anderson & Ward, 1976). Haber (1977) and his colleagues have suggested that fibre-depleted foods result in an abnormally rapid absorption of carbohydrate and an excessive stimulation of insulin secretion which could eventually lead to diabetes. This hypothesis is based on a study of apples which were fed in differing forms, apple juice which is devoid of fibre, apple puree, and whole apple. They found that the juice could be consumed 11 times faster than intact apples and that pureed apples could be eaten four times faster than whole apples. With the rate of ingestion equal, juice was significantly less satisfying than puree and similarly puree was less satisfying than whole apple. The plasma glucose rose to similar levels after each of the three meals. However, there was a

striking rebound found in the blood glucose after juice and to a less extent after puree. This phenomenon was not seen with the whole apples. Serum insulins rose to a higher concentration after juice and puree than after apples. This means that the removal of the fibre from food and also its physical disruption can result in faster and easier digestion, and decreased satiety and that it alters glucose homeostasis and insulin secretion.

Fibre in the colon

The colon can be regarded as two organs, the right side being a fermenter in which there is bacterial activity and also absorption of water, electrolytes and organic substances. Such absorption converts the liquid coming from the ileum into the solid concentrate constituting the stool. The left side of the colon is a conserver of continence through circular muscle contraction. Fibre in the colon may act by forming a supporting matrix which provides surfaces or in trapping bacteria within the interstices of the fibre. In this environment bacteria and intestinal contents inter-react. Fibre may alter the metabolism of compounds in the colon through bacteria behaving differently when attached to a fibre matrix than when they are in free solution. Metabolic products may be adsorbed to the fibre or the absorption from that product from the lumen being facilitated by the chemical change.

The chemical nature of the metabolic products may well be determined by the presence of fibre. It has been shown by Ershoff (1972) that detergents when fed to rats can be toxic. This toxicity can be protected against by the presence of fibre. Different fibres differ in their protective ability. Cyclamate, the artificial sweetener, is a highly polar compound which is not readily absorbed from the intestine. In the caecum, cyclamate is converted to cyclohexylamine and other products. These products are believed to be toxic, but such toxicity is prevented if fibre is added to the diet.

It is conceivable that fibre in the caecum may bring order into caecal metabolism and influence the fate of compounds.

Effect of fibre on stool weight

The rural African who eats a high-fibre-containing diet passes approximately 500 g of stool per day. In contrast, an individual who eats a low-fibre-containing diet passes a small stool of approximately 80 g per day.

Bran is a laxative whose property has been known since early times. In 1936 Williams & Olmstedt produced a table of the ability of various plant sources to increase stool weight. Agar agar, carrot, cabbage and sugar-beet pulp were the most effective plant sources. There was a 20-fold difference between the capacity to bind water of cotton-seed wholes, which was the least effective influence on stool weight, and of the most effective - agar agar. In 1945 Hoppert & Clark showed that bran and cabbage had the most consistent and favourably laxative effect whereas certain vegetables, eg lettuce, gave less pronounced effects. It was suggested by Hoppert & Clark that the laxative properties of food could be evaluated as a result of physiological studies and not on the basis of the crude-fibre values. McConnell and his colleagues (1974) showed that it is possible to tabulate fruit and vegetable as water absorbers. However, more recently Cummings and his colleagues (1978) have suggested that it is the pentose fraction of the fibrous material which is most important in influencing the stool size. However, water-holding capacity of cereal bran is important. Coarse bran is much more effective than fine bran because of its greater water-holding capacity (Kirwan *et al.*, 1974).

The bulking action of dietary fibre will have the effect of diluting colonic contents. This means that the biological effects of compounds in the stool will be diluted as a result.

The effect of fibre on transit time

Transit time is the time taken for the passage of materials from the mouth to anus. The transit time varies considerably from person to person and even in any one person the transit time is not constant. The transit time is influenced by the method which is used to measure the transit time, of which specific gravity is very important. It may well be that changes in stool characteristics and specific gravity may also influence the transit time of a marker of constant specific gravity. One definition of constipation is a delay in the overall transit time. Such a delay is always in the descending colon. The prolonged form of transit time may well be in excess of four, five or even ten days. A normal transit time may be within 24 and 48 hours. There is a differential rate of flow of liquid and solid phases through the gastrointestinal tract. This of course makes the estimation of transit time even more complicated.

The effect of fibre on electrolyte excretion

Because of the cation-exchange properties of fibre there is an enhanced faecal-electrolyte excretion following the addition of fibre to the diet. This has been raised as a possible source of danger in increasing the fibre content of the diet.

This may not be a problem in the Western diet with its range of constituents. A high-fibre-containing diet has however been shown to be a source of malnutrition of trace elements in Iran (Reinhold *et al.*, 1973).

Fibre and serum lipids

This is one of the more intriguing aspects of fibre. It is known that fibre on its own can protect experimental animals against the atherogenic effects of certain fatty diets. Most diets used to develop atheroma in animals are fibre free. Vegetarians have a low serum cholesterol and a lower rate of coronary heart disease than meat eaters in the same society. However, those fibrous materials which have been shown to be substantial adsorbers of bile acids have yet to prove to be highly effective in reducing the serum cholesterol. Bile acids are adsorbed to fibre and bile acids are strongly adsorbed to fibres in the stool. If bran is added to the diet of human subjects there is no effect on the serum cholesterol. However, pectin and pectin-containing fibres can reduce the serum cholesterol (Story & Kritchevsky, 1976; Kay & Truswell, 1977).

The place of fibre in human nutrition

It is not known whether the long-term ingestion of fibre has any effect on preventing appendicitis, carcinoma of the colon and diverticular disease and haemorrhoids. There are indications that vegetarians have a reduced risk of coronary artery disease and diverticular disease. It is also clear now that the best treatment of constipation or faecal stasis in diverticular disease, simple constipation, ulcerative colitis and haemorrhoids is by using fibre. It is worthwhile getting the patient to eat wholemeal bread and to eat coarse bran making it palatable with milk and either raisins or cooked fruit to modify its texture. There are commercially available high-bran-containing preparations, eg All Bran. My practice is to suggest that the patient takes a handful of bran per day for the first week, and two handfuls thereafter. There may well prove to be advantages for pectin-containing substances in the diet which may influence cholesterol metabolism and absorption from the small intestine. This latter property may prove to be valuable in the control of diabetes and also in treating the dumping syndrome which can complicate peptic-ulcer surgery.

A contrary indication to enhancing the fibre content of the diet is known obstruction of the intestine, as in adhesions. Volvulus is said to be more common in countries whose diet habitually has a high fibre content.

References

Alvarez, W.C. (1949): *An introduction to gastroenterology*, 4th edn. London: Heineman.

Anon (1977): *Lancet* 2, 337-338.

Burkitt, D.P. (1973): *Proc. Nutr. Soc.* 32, 145.

Cleave, T.L., Campbell, G.D. & Painter, N.S. (1966): *Diabetes, coronary thrombosis and the saccharine disease.* Bristol: John Wright.

Cummings, J.H. (1975): In *Fiber in human nutrition,* ed G.A. Spiller & R.J. Amen. New York: Plenum Press.

Cummings, J.H., Southgate, D.A.T., Branch, W., Houston, H., Jenkins, D.J.A. & James, W.P.T. (1978): *Lancet* 1, 5-9.

Eastwood, M.A. & Hamilton, D. (1968): *Biochem. Biophys. Acta* 152, 165.

Eastwood, M.A. & Mitchell, W.D. (1976): In *Fiber in human nutrition,* ed G.A. Spiller & R.J. Amen. New York: Plenum Press.

Ershoff, B.H. (1972): *Proc. Soc. Exp. Biol. Med.* 141, 857.

Haber, G.R., Heaton, K.W., Murphy, D. & Burroughs, L.F. (1977): *Lancet* 2, 679.

Hoppert, C.A. & Clark, A.J. (1945): *J. Am. Diet. Ass.* 21, 157.

Jenkins, D.J.A., Leeds, A.R.L., Rassull, M.A., Cochet, B. & Alberti, G.M.M. (1977): *Ann. Int. Med.* 86, 20.

Kay, R.M. & Truswell, A.S. (1977): *Br. J. Nutr.* 37, 227.

Kiehm, T.G., Anderson, J.W. & Ward, K. (1976): *Am. J. Clin. Nutr.* 29, 895.

Kirwan, W.O., Smith, A.N., McConnell, A.A., Mitchell, W.D. & Eastwood, M.A. (1974): *Br. Med. J.* 2, 187.

Kritchevsky, D. (1964): *J. Atheroscler. Res.* 4, 103.

McCance, R.A. & Widdowson, E.M. (1955): *Lancet* 2, 205.

McConnell, A.A., Eastwood, M.A. & Mitchell, W.D. (1974): *J. Sci. Fd Agric.* 25, 1457.

Malhotra, S.L. (1968): *Br. Heart J.* 30, 303.

Moore, J.H. (1967): *Br. J. Nutr.* 21, 207.

Painter, N.S. (1975): *Diverticular disease of the colon.* London: Heineman.

Portman, O.W. (1960): *Am. J. Clin. Nutr.* 8, 462.

Rees, D.A. (1967): *The shapes of molecules, carbohydrate polymers.* Edinburgh: Oliver and Boyd.

Reinhold, J.G., Nars, K., Lahimgarzadeh, A. & Hedayati, H. (1973): *Lancet* 1, 283.

Southgate, D.A.T. (1976): In *Fiber in human nutrition,* ed G.A. Spiller & R.J. Amen. New York: Plenum Press.

Story, J.A. & Kritchevsky, D. (1976): In *Fiber in human nutrition,* ed G.A. Spiller & R.J. Amen. New York: Plenum Press.

Trowell, H.C. (1972): *Lancet* 1, 503.

Trowell, H.C. (1973): *Proc. Nutr. Soc.* 32, 151.

Williams, R.D. & Olmsted, W.H. (1936): *J. Nutr.* 2, 433.

Van Soest, P.J. & McQueen, R.W. (1973): *Proc. Nutr. Soc.* 32, 123.

6

Sucrose

Ian Macdonald.

Introduction

Sweetness is a sensation that has been acceptable to man since he first ate fruit and honey. This desire for sweetness led to the cultivation of plants especially for their ability to produce sweetness, and the most acceptable of these natural sweet compounds is sucrose. This is fortunate as not only is sucrose relatively cheap to produce but it has many properties that make it very useful as a food ingredient (Table 1).

Table 1. Properties of sucrose as a food ingredient

Increases:	Sweetness Osmotic pressure Viscosity Boiling point
Enhances:	Flavour Appearance – improved lustre, clarity and gloss
Other properties:	Provides bulk ('body') Affects solubility of ingredients Has solvent properties Imparts plasticity Assists emulsification Can be fermented Can be crystallized Penetrates other ingredients, eg fruit and vegetables

Composition

Sucrose, commonly referred to simply as 'sugar', is a dissacharide composed of glucose and fructose. In solution it is the mode of carbohydrate transport in plants and squeezing the sap from the stem of the sugar cane is one of the two common sources of sucrose. The other common source, and the only one in the UK, is sugar beet where it is part of the storage carbohydrate of the plant.

Consumption

The consumption of sucrose in the UK has been rising for the past 130 years or so[10], but now seems to have reached a peak and it may even be falling (Fig. 1) perhaps, in part, due to competition from other natural sweetners such as glucose syrups and fructose syrups. The proportion of sucrose that is used in various foods in the UK is seen in Fig. 2.

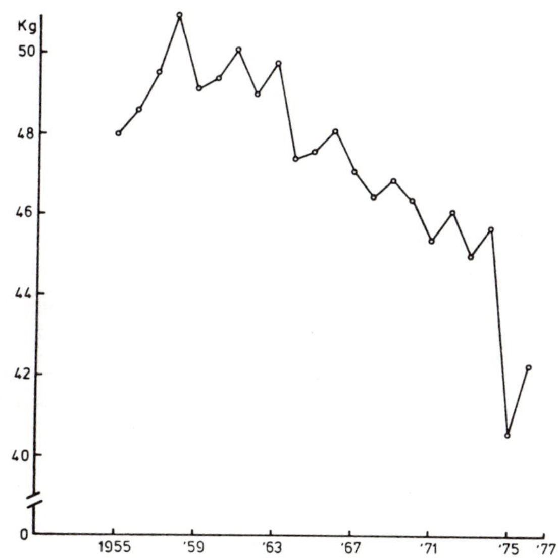

Fig. 1. Refined sucrose consumption in UK (kg per head per annum). From *Trade and Industry* 1976: 596

Sucrose in the body

Digestion

Though some slight hydrolysis of sucrose might occur in the acid environment of the stomach, most of the breakdown of sucrose to glucose and fructose occurs in the brush border of the intestine, notably in its upper part. Activity of the enzyme sucrase is significantly higher on a sucrose diet than on a glucose diet, and it has been shown that fructose is the active principle in the induction of sucrase[22].

Glucose passes through the gut wall by means of 'active' transport, a system which is sodium-dependent[6]. This 'active' transport is necessary to prevent the osmotic effects seen when monosaccharides which are absorbed passively (ie down a concentration gradient) are taken in large quantities. The colic and diarrhoea produced by, for example, a large amount of sorbitol or xylitol, are evidence that water is being drawn into the intestinal lumen at a faster rate than sugar is being absorbed.

Fructose transport across the intestinal wall is 'facilitated', in that it goes across faster than can be accounted for by passive diffusion, and yet there is no

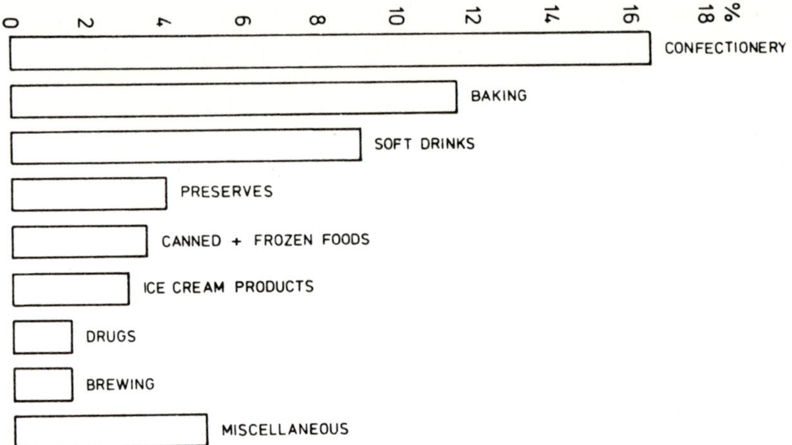

Fig. 2. Properties of sucrose used in various foods etc. in six months ending March, 1977 in the UK (Personal communication)

evidence that the process is active[8]. It is of interest to note that 70 g fructose by mouth will give rise to abdominal discomfort and perhaps diarrhoea in an adult, whereas 200 g sucrose, containing nearly 100 g fructose, does not result in any abdominal discomfort.

Some of the fructose is converted in the intestinal mucosa to glucose, but the exact proportion is uncertain as conversions from 30 to 70 per cent have been reported in man[4]. Serum fructose levels are higher in man when given in sucrose than when given in an equal mixture of glucose and fructose, and the high concentration of fructose in the brush border after hydrolysis of sucrose may facilitate absorption by giving rise to a steeper concentration gradient of fructose[17].

Sucrose, when given intravenously, is excreted unchanged in the urine as there is no sucrase in the body other than that in the gut wall.

Metabolic fate of sucrose

Since sucrose is absorbed as the monosaccharides glucose and fructose, the ultimate fate of sucrose is that of these two constituent monosaccharides. Figs 3 and 4 show in outline the end-products of glucose and fructose metabolism, where it can be seen that glucose may be stored as glycogen, converted to body

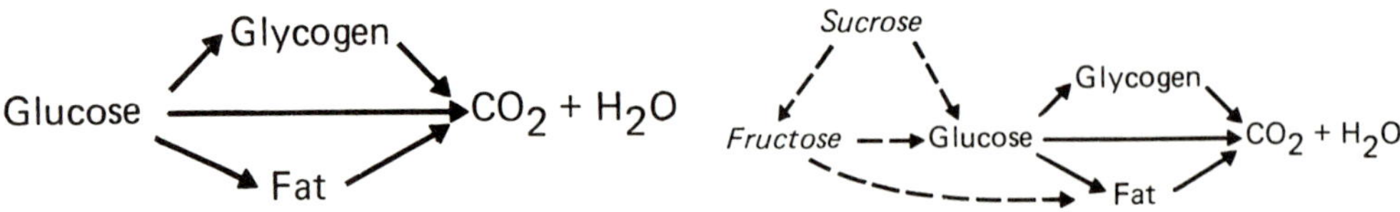

Fig. 3. Metabolic fates of glucose

Fig. 4. Metabolic fates of sucrose

fat or catabolised to carbon dioxide and water with energy as the vital component. Fructose can be converted to glucose either in the gut wall or. mainly, in the liver and hence shares the fate of glucose, or it can be converted by the liver to triglyceride and this lipid can be stored in the adipose tissue.

The breakdown of glucose to the trioses di-hydroxyacetone phosphate and glyceraldehyde-phosphate is rate-limiting, but the comparable breakdown of fructose is not rate-limiting and this may lead to clinical disturbances. In man, fructose disappears from the circulation twice as fast as glucose.

Among the metabolic disturbances that may result from consuming a single large amount of fructose as such or as sucrose are[27]:

Lactic acidosis. This is more likely to occur when the subject has liver disease, and would also exacerbate a pre-existing acidosis.

Hyperuricaemia. The rapid phosphorylation of fructose decreases the concentration of ATP, with a consequent depletion of adenine nucleotides in the liver and formation of adenosine and inosine, and hence uric acid.

Clinical conditions and sucrose consumption

Dental caries

Caries is an infectious disease which requires not only an organism – *Streptococcus mutans* – but an environment that is conducive to the growth of the organism. Part of the environment is carbohydrate – in particular, sucrose. The organism converts carbohydrates into a plaque which means that the organisms and their by-products such as acid are kept in close, constant contact with the enamel, which eventually is broken down and the dentine exposed and then decalcified.

In animals, sucrose has been found to be the most cariogenic of the carbohydrates and it is known that people with fructose intolerance, and who therefore do not consume fructose in any form, have less dental caries than average. It seems that the consumption, by man, of 'sticky' sucrose products between meals increases the extent of dental caries[19].

Obesity

There seems to be a widespread impression that sucrose is more likely to cause obesity than any other single item in the diet. This impression is not supported by any scientific evidence; the energy the body derives from sucrose is no different to that from other dietary sources, in fact, fat contains, per unit weight, more than twice as much energy as sucrose. That sucrose consumption is a common cause of obesity may well be true, not because it contains more energy, but because more of it is eaten than is metabolically desirable. This is a reflection of the palatability of sucrose, and furthermore dietary advice tends to recommend that the amount of sucrose consumed by the slimmer be reduced because its reduced intake would offset an indulgence and its omission would, furthermore, be unlikely to result in any nutritional deficiency. The acceptance that dietary carbohydrate may be converted to body fat has long been known[12], especially in the live-stock trade, though the reverse is not within the capability of the body. It is assumed that all dietary carbohydrates which are iso-energetic, as determined in a bomb calorimeter, are also metabolically iso-energetic. This may not be so[16].

Diabetes

Obesity or over-weight in a middle-aged adult may give rise to the so-called 'maturity-onset' diabetes, a condition in which there is not only no absence of insulin but, in fact, the reverse is true. However, it would appear that in this condition there is a degree of 'insulin resistance' in that more insulin is required to handle a fixed amount of glucose than in a healthy person. Inasmuch as any food which is over-consumed can result in this kind of diabetes, sucrose is no different from the rest. In fact, sucrose by mouth gives rise to about half the insulin output compared to a similar load of glucose[25].

There is some suggestion from animal experiments that a high sucrose, compared with glucose, intake increases the incidence of the insulin-deficient type of diabetes[3], but attempts to associate diabetes in man with a high sucrose intake have failed[26].

There are, however, some good reasons why glucose is to be preferred to sucrose in the treatment of diabetic acidosis. Sucrose raises pyruvate and lactate levels in the blood whereas glucose reduces these levels[18] and in such an acidosis it is preferable that those substances which may be raised are not further elevated. Sucrose contains fructose and in diabetic acidosis this additional fructose would be undesirable. Sucrose therefore has no place in the treatment of diabetic acidosis – neither does fructose.

Coronary artery disease

There is widespread belief that sucrose predisposes to coronary artery disease and some official pronouncements lend support to this. However, the evidence to support this view is incomplete and though carbohydrates as a group may in some persons pre-dispose to coronary artery disease there is only presumptive evidence that sucrose is more malevolent in this respect.

If the person is a maturity-onset diabetic who is overweight, and therefore prone to develop ischaemic heart disease, then sucrose intake should be reduced – not because of sucrose *per se* but because sucrose should form part of a generalised reduction in energy intake.

Hyperlipidaemia

In one type of hyperlipidaemia (IV) the level of triglycerides in fasting serum is raised above normal and these triglycerides are endogenous in that they are made in the liver largely from carbohydrate in the diet. In those patients who have this lipid abnormality (13 per cent of the adult male population)[23] an increase in the proportion of carbohydrate in the diet will lead to an increase in the fasting serum triglyceride level and vice versa[7]. There is experimental evidence in man that an unusually high intake of sucrose will cause this triglyceride level to be greater than after a corresponding intake of glucose, or its polymer, starch[15]. There is also suggestive evidence that if the high-carbohydrate diet is persisted in, then the initial raised level of serum triglyceride will drop, but perhaps not to the level found before the increased carbohydrate consumption[2]. It is not known whether with sucrose the final level would be higher than with starch. There is some evidence to show that when glucose replaces sucrose in the diet there is a fall in the level of endogenous triglyceride in the serum and that this fall is greater in those whose level of triglyceride was high[21].

The capacity of sucrose to increase the level of endogenous triglyceride in the serum is due to the fructose moeity in its molecule, because fructose given with glucose has a similar effect, an effect not seen with glucose alone.

Sucrose probably has no effect on serum cholesterol levels. The slight increase in serum cholesterol which accompanies hypertriglyceridaemia is due to a small quantity of cholesterol present in the very-low-density lipoprotein fraction which is mainly responsible for triglyceride transport.

Effects of sucrose in the diet

Relationship with dietary fat

It is known that the amount and type of carbohydrate in the diet may, in some people, increase the level of triglyceride in the fasting serum. However, food consists of substances other than carbohydrate and studies on the effects of the amount and type of fat in the diet have shown that these effects can override those produced by carbohydrate. The rise in fasting serum triglyceride concentration that can occur after switching to a high-sucrose diet can be exaggerated by the partial substitution of sucrose by saturated fat, and can be negated by the partial substitution of sucrose by polyunsaturated fat[14]. It thus seems that the amount and type of fat in the diet may be as influential on fasting serum triglyceride levels as the amount and type of carbohydrate. It has been shown, both in healthy men and in those who have had a coronary thrombosis, that the triglyceridaemic effects of sucrose can be prevented by the addition of corn oil to the diet[1].

Relationship with dietary protein

Fructose, and therefore indirectly sucrose, can influence protein absorption in that, compared with glucose, it increases the absorption of leucine and lysine[20]. On the other hand the rate of recovery of serum albumin levels in protein-deficient animals is slower with sucrose in the diet than with starch[9].

The glucose moeity of sucrose, in man, impairs the rate of absorption of glycine and vice versa[5]. Leucine also inhibits the absorption of glucose. Thus it is unwise to consider any food substance in isolation because it effects and is affected by other substances present in the food.

Relationship with sex of the consumer

The metabolic effects of any nutrient are affected by both the physiological and pathological state of the consumer as earlier reference to 'carbohydrate-sensitive' persons shows. It has also been found that the metabolic response to fructose and sucrose depends on the gender of the consumer. With diets high in sucrose young women, unlike men of a comparable age group, do not have an increase in fasting serum triglyceride concentration. In post-menopausal women the effect is similar to that of the men[13]. Sucrose taken at the same time as an oestrogen-progestagen oral contraceptive will produce a lipid response similar to that seen in males[24] and it is known that in pregnancy the serum triglyceride and cholesterol levels are raised, though it is not known whether sucrose would exaggerate these levels. It is not known which hormone or hormones is responsible for these variable metabolic reactions to fructose, though it has been reported that in young women the enzyme lipoprotein lipase which removes the trigycerides from serum is more effective than in men[11]. The difference in response to fructose may, therefore, not reflect a difference in the rate of conversion of fructose to triglyceride so much as a difference in the clearance of the triglyceride so formed.

Some acute effects after ingestion of sucrose
When sucrose in water is taken after an overnight fast the differences between this carbohydrate and others can give clues to the metabolic differences between the carbohydrates consumed. The mean level of blood glucose after taking sucrose by mouth is about the same as that seen after taking glucose and the response is not dose-related. The serum insulin elevation, on the other hand, is twice as much with glucose as with sucrose (because fructose does not stimulate insulin release) and the insulin levels are dose-related.

Sucrose and performance in sport
From the findings above where sucrose raises the blood levels of lactate and pyruvate, it would seem that it would be preferable to take glucose in preference in those sports of moderate duration where carbohydrate 'topping-up' is useful. However, as sucrose is a disaccharide, weight-for-weight it exerts about half the osmotic pressure of glucose and this must be considered in terms of palatibility and abdominal discomfort due to possible delay in stomach emptying with a raised osmotic pressure in the gastric contents. The sweetness of sucrose is more acceptable than that of glucose and this would make sucrose more palatable.

Though the insulin output following ingestion of sucrose is half that occurring after an equal quantity of glucose, the hypoglycaemia following the ingestion of carbohydrates in the fasting state seems to be more marked after sucrose.

As expected, weight-for-weight the serum fructose levels after sucrose ingestion are about half those seen after fructose alone. The lactate and pyruvate levels do not change and even fall after ingesting glucose, but after sucrose they always rise and this rise seems to be greater than that which follows ingestion of an equal weight of fructose. Sucrose, because of its fructose component, causes an elevation of blood uric acid and for this reason it would be wise to restrict sucrose or fructose intake in those persons who have gout.

Conclusions

Sucrose has a different effect on the metabolism from that of glucose or even the disaccharide of glucose, namely maltose. To a large extent this difference is due to the fructose moeity of sucrose. Whether, apart from dental caries, the differences in metabolic response to sucrose, compared to glucose or its polymers, are detrimental to the well-being of the consumer is not known with any degree of certainty and before definitive statements can be made about the effects of sucrose on health more needs to be discovered. In view of the increasing production and utilization of fructose syrups which contain fructose and glucose (cf honey) the assessment of the long-term effects of fructose ingestion in man would seem to be relevant.

References

1. Antar, M.A., Little, J.A., Lucas, P., Buckley, G.C. & Csima, A. (1970): *Atheroscl.* **11**, 191.
2. Antonis, A. & Bersohn, I. (1961): *Lancet* **1**, 3.
3. Cohen, A.M. & Teitelbaum, A. (1964): *Am. J. Physiol.* **206**, 1.

4. Cook, G.C. (1969): *Clin. Sci.* **37**, 675.
5. Cook, G.C. (1971): *J. Physiol.* (Lond.) **217**, 61.
6. Crane, R.K. (1977): *Internat. Rev. Physiol.* **12**, 325.
7. Fredrickson, D.S., Levy, R.I. & Lees, R.S. (1967): *New Engl. J. Med.* **276**, 34, 94, 148, 215 and 273.
8. Gracey, M., Burke, V. & Oshin, A. (1972): *Biochem. Biophys. Acta* **266**, 397.
9. Grimble, R.F. (1975): *Nutr. Rep. Internat.* **12**, 331.
10. Hollingsworth, D.F. & Greaves, J.P. (1967): *Am. J. Clin. Nutr.* **20**, 65.
11. Kekki, M. & Nikkila, E.A. (1971): *Metabolism* **20**, 878.
12. Lawes, J.B. & Gilbert, J.H. (1852): *Br. Ass. Adv. Sci. Rep.* 323.
13. Macdonald, I. (1966): *Am. J. Clin. Nutr.* **20**, 345.
14. Macdonald, I. (1972): *Clin. Sci.* **43**, 265.
15. Macdonald, I. & Braithwaite, D.M. (1964): *Clin. Sci.* **27**, 23.
16. Macdonald, I. & Grenby, T. (1979): *Proc. Nutr. Soc.* **38**, 30A.
17. Macdonald, I. & Turner, L.J. (1968): *Lancet* **1**, 841.
18. Macdonald, I., Keyser, A., & Pacy, D. (1978): *Am. J. Clin. Nutr.* **31**, 1305.
19. Makinen, K.K. (1974): In *Sugars in nutrition,* ed Sipple, H.L. & K.W. McNutt, p. 645. New York: Academic press.
20. Reiser, S. & Hallfrisch, J. (1977): *J. Nutr.* **107**, 767.
21. Roberts, A.M. (1973): *Lancet* **1**, 1201.
22. Rosenweig, N.S. & Herman, R.H. (1968): *J. Clin. Invest.* **47**, 2253.
23. Stone, M.C. & Dick, T.B.S. (1973): *Br. Heart. J.* **35**, 954.
24. Stovin, V. & Macdonald, I. (1975): *Proc. Nutr. Soc.* **34**, 55A.
25. Thompson, R.G., Hayford, J.T. & Danney, M.M. (1978): *Diabetes* **27**, 1020.
26. West, M.K. (1975): *Nutr. Rev.* **33**, 193.
27. Woods, H.F. & Alberti, K.G.M.M. (1972): *Lancet* **2**, 1354.

Bibliography

Berdanier, C.D. Editor (1976): *Carbohydrate metabolism.* London: John Wiley.
Macdonald, I. Editor (1973): *Effect of carbohydrates on lipid metabolism.* Basel: Karger.
Sipple, H.L. & McNutt, K.W. Editors (1974): *Sugars in nutrition.* New York: Academic Press.
Yudkin, J., Edelman, J. & Hough, L. Editors (1971): *Sugar.* London: Butterworth.

7
Obesity

Margaret Ashwell, Merril Durrant, Penelope Warwick and J. S. Garrow.

Introduction

Obesity and its medical complications have been recognised for several centuries. The condition was described by Hippocrates, and Socrates is said to have danced every morning in order to keep thin. The Romans invented the vomitorium so that people who had eaten to excess could make themselves sick afterwards and not gain weight as a result of their gluttony. Obesity has been depicted in art through the ages both as representing prosperity and affluence, and as one of the deadly sins – greed. Brillat Savarin (1889) wrote that any cure for obesity must begin with three precepts: discretion in eating, moderation in sleeping, and exercise on foot or horseback. This view was reiterated by von Noorden in 1900. In his book 'Die Fettsucht' he described the state of obesity as a result of positive energy balance, that is, over-eating or under-exercising.

The contemporary importance of obesity and its medical complications is well reviewed in the joint publication from the Department of Health & Social Security and the Medical Research Council (1976). To quote from the first paragraph: 'We are unanimous in our belief that obesity is a hazard to health and a detriment to well-being. It is common enough to constitute one of the most important medical and public health problems of our time, whether we judge importance by a shorter expectation of life, increased morbidity, or cost to the community in terms of both money and anxiety.'

The prevalence of obesity in the United Kingdom

All the evidence on the prevalence of obesity in adults in this country is based on measurement of body weight in relation to age and height. The drawback of this method of assessment is that no index of weight and height alone can differentiate overweight caused by an excess of fat (ie obesity) from overweight caused by an excess of muscle. Bearing this in mind, the reader is referred to Tables 1 & 2 which summarise the mean values for the weight-height index (W/H^2) of men and women in different surveys in the UK during the last 50 years. The figures in these tables confirm the increase in the value of W/H^2 (and therefore probably obesity) with age in both sexes and show that there has been a small increase since the wartime surveys of 1943.

Table 1. Mean values for the weight-height index (W/H^2) of men in different surveys undertaken in the UK during the last 50 years (weight in kg; height in metres)

Year of survey	Group	Age (yrs) 20-25 W/H^2	35-40 W/H^2	55-60 W/H^2	Reference
1930	National	21.3	22.8	23.3	Khosla & Lowe (1968)
1943	National	21.8	22.7	24.6	Khosla & Lowe (1968)
1960	Birmingham	22.8	24.9	24.9	Khosla & Lowe (1968)
1965	Port Talbot	24.3	26.2	26.2	Khosla & Lowe (1968)
1969	Directors	—	25.6*	26.2	Richardson & Pincherle (1969)
1971	BP Employees	22.5	24.3†	25.4‡	Montegriffo (1971)
1974	Richmond§	22.6	24.9	24.7	Baird *et al.* (1974)

* Middle age group, 35-44 years; upper age group, 55-64 years †Age group, 30-39 years
‡ Age group, 50-59 years § Lower age group, 15-29 years, middle, 30-49 years; upper 50-65 years

Mean values of W/H^2 for different populations do not give information about the proportion of individuals who are overweight, but this is always a very difficult thing to do because the number of overweight people depends entirely on the definition of 'overweight'. If the middle of the medium-frame weights for heights given by the build and blood pressure study of the Chicago Society of Actuaries (1959) is taken to be ideal weight, and overweight is defined as a weight which is more than 10 per cent above ideal weight, then 37 per cent of the men and 36.5 per cent of the women in the UK are overweight (Baird *et al.*, 1974).

Table 2. Mean values for the weight-height index (W/H^2) of women in three surveys (weight in kg; height in metres)

Year of survey	Group	Young adult* W/H^2	Early middle age† W/H^2	Late middle age‡ W/H^2	Reference
1943	National	20.7	22.5	23.6	Khosla & Lowe (1968)
1971	BP employees	21.6	22.9	25.9	Montegriffo (1971)
1974	Richmond	21.6	23.7	25.1	Baird *et al.* (1974)

*Young, 20-25 or 29-30 years † Early middle age, 30-49 or 35-40 years ‡ Late middle age 50-65 or 50-60 years

Energy balance

Although there is much discussion about the relative roles that genes and environment play in the development of obesity (see Ashwell, 1975), the basic energy-balance equation has yet to be disproved. This equation says, that if energy intake exceeds energy output, the excess energy will be stored by the body. In this review, we will start by considering the nature of these energy stores and their relationship to the natural history and treatment of obesity. Then we will take a closer look at the 'energy intake' side of the equation and see whether or not obese people differ from lean people in the way in which they regulate their energy intake. Finally, we will look at the 'energy output' side of the equation and explore the differences between obese and lean people.

Energy stores

The relationship of energy stores to body composition is clearly shown in Fig. 1*a* & *b* (Garrow, 1978*a*). Figure 1*a* shows the situation in a normal 70 kg man. Although water is the main component of body weight, it contributes nothing to energy stores. The greatest proportion of energy stores is derived from the adipose tissue (total weight = 18 kg, total energy = 527 MJ, 126 Mcal). The

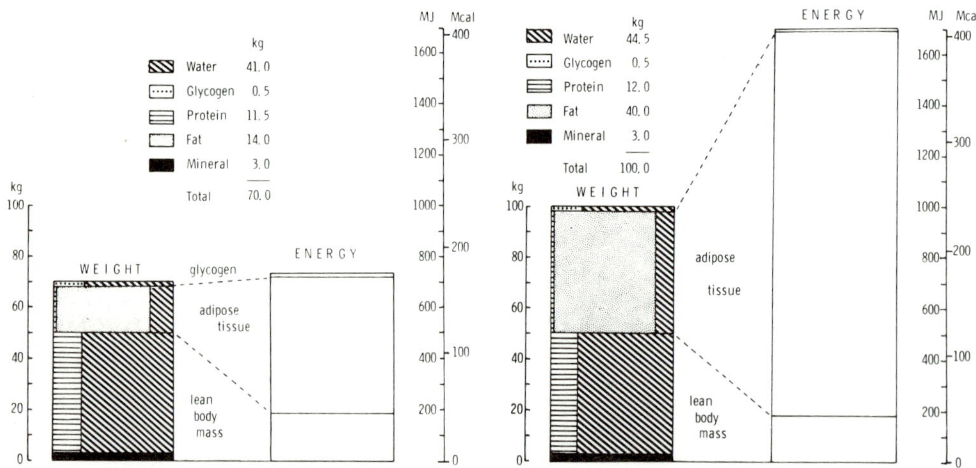

Fig. 1a. The body composition of a normal adult male who weighs 70 kg. Left: the approximate composition of lean body mass and adipose tissue in terms of the weight of water, protein, fat and mineral; right: the equivalent energy values of these components. The glycogen-water pool is assumed to be 2 kg (From J.S. Garrow, *Energy balance in man,* by permission of North Holland Publishing)

Fig. 1b. The body composition of an obese adult male who weighs 100 kg. The lean body mass and glycogen pool have been assumed to be similar to that of the subject shown in Fig. 1a. The extra weight is due to an extra 30 kg of adipose tissue, which has increased the energy stores by approximately 1000 MJ (From J.S. Garrow, *Energy balance in man,* by permission of North Holland Publishing)

glycogen-water pool which is assumed to be 2 kg (0.5 kg glycogen and 1.5 kg water) represents a minor energy store (total energy = 8.37 MJ, 2000 kcal). Figure 1*b* shows that if the hypothetical subject in Fig. 1*a* becomes obese by the acquisition of an extra 30 kg adipose tissue, then it is even more obvious that the vast proportion of his energy stores is found as adipose tissue.

In this section we will discuss first the way in which the total amount of adipose tissue (fat) in the body can be measured and the methods used to measure the size of the individual fat cells. After this, we will consider the relevance of adipose tissue cellularity to the natural history and the treatment of obesity.

The measurement of total body fat

Several methods have been used to measure total body fat in man; see Garrow (1978*a*) for a full description of methods and limitations. Briefly, the simplest method, ie that of measuring skinfold thicknesses and deriving total fat from equations, is the one which is least accurate when it is used for the obese. The most accurate methods, which determine fat from body density or indirectly from measurements of body water, are unfortunately the ones which require expensive and specialised apparatus.

Total fat is made up of internal (visceral) and external (subcutaneous) fat. Very few studies have investigated the relative proportions of these components in normal-weight subjects, let alone in obese ones. Estimates of the proportion of internal fat to total fat range from 11 per cent to 42 per cent for lean subjects. Subcutaneous fat distribution has been studied more extensively (see Ashwell *et al.*, 1978*a* for a review of the literature).

The measurement of fat cell size

Adipocytes (fat cells), with diameters ranging up to 150 μm, are the largest cells found anywhere in the body. Next to blood cells, they are perhaps the easiest cells to study in man, since an adipose tissue biopsy can be performed with minor discomfort to the patient. Yields of up to 500 mg can be obtained with a simple needle biopsy (see Fig. 2).

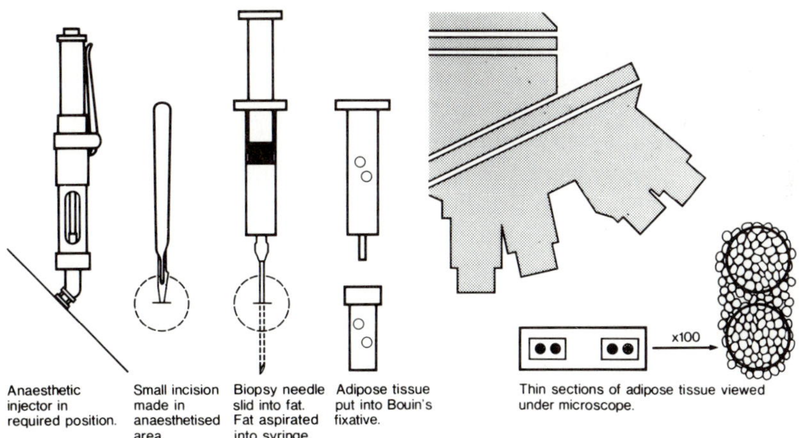

Fig. 2. Human fat biopsy technique and histological measurement of the fat cell size

During the last decade, a lot of attention has been focussed on fat cell size and its relevance to obesity. Table 3 summarises the various methods of measurement (see Gurr & Kirtland (1978) or Björntorp (1978) for further details).

It has been the practice in our own laboratory to measure cell size from wax embedded sections (Fig. 2); Fig. 3*a* - *f* shows samples of adipose tissue taken with a biopsy needle from three sites in the same patient before and after a

Table 3. Measurement of fat cell size

Method	Advantages	Disadvantages
Isolated cell methods		
(a) Fixed cells Osmium tetroxide fixation, dispersed cells counted electronically, cell size derived from number and lipid weight.	Automated	Expensive. No measure of 'in situ' arrangement of cells.
(b) Unfixed cells Collagenase dispersion, microscopic (± photographic) measurement of diameters.	Direct measurement of diameters	Cell breakage? Time consuming. No 'in situ' information.
Fixed whole tissue methods		
(a) Frozen-cut sections Brief fixation, frozen thick sections cut, microscopic (± photographic) measurement of diameters.	Cheap. Immediate results. 'In situ' information.	Time consuming. Correction factors needed?
(b) Wax-embedded sections Fixation, embedding in wax, thin sections cut, microscopic (± photographic) examination – measurement of diameters or counting of cells in fixed area.	Cheap and quick (if routine service available). Not laborious. 'In-situ' information.	Correction factors needed.

weight loss of 34.2 kg. These photomicrographs show not only the regional variation in cell size that exists before weight reduction, but show also the decrease in cell size at all sites after weight loss.

The estimation of total fat cell number

Since it is possible to measure the total amount of fat and the size of the individual fat cells, it should theoretically be possible to calculate the total number of fat cells in the body by dividing total fat by average fat cell mass. This has been done many times, and much significance has been attached to measurement of fat cell number (FCN) in obesity, but there is currently controversy about the accuracy of such estimates.

First the calculation of FCN assumes that the fat cells measured in a biopsy are typical of the fat cells throughout the body. This is certainly not the case: internal fat cells which cannot be sampled by needle biopsy are usually smaller than subcutaneous fat cells and even subcutaneous fat cells can show wide variations in size in some individuals (see Fig. 3). Secondly, all methods of fat cell sizing can only measure lipid-containing cells. There is now evidence that adipose tissue has non-lipid-containing precursor cells which would not be counted by any of the existing methods (see Ashwell, 1978). Thirdly, some of the indirect methods used to calculate body fat can be rather misleading when they are used before and after weight loss or gain, since water and fat are not always lost or gained in constant proportions. The subsequent calculations of FCN before and after weight loss or gain would therefore also be misleading.

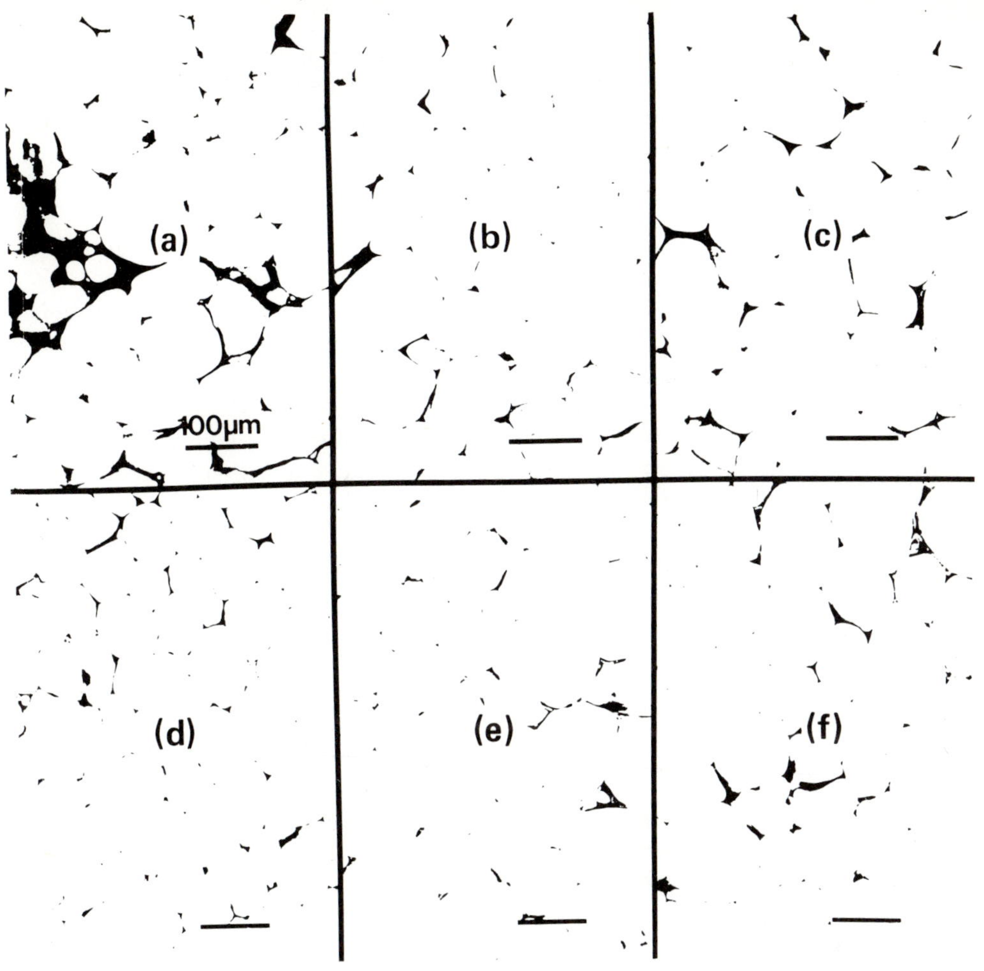

Fig. 3. Photomicrographs of adipose tissue obtained by needle biopsy from three subcutaneous sites in a patient who reduced her weight from 92.7 kg. to 58.5 kg. Scale marker = 100 μM
(a) shows adipose tissue from the lateral arm *before* weight reduction.Mean fat cell diameter (±s.d.) = 110±15.5μM, mean fat cell mass = 0.68μg.
(b) shows adipose tissue from the abdomen *before* weight reduction. Mean fat cell diameter (±s.d.) = 113.8±15.8μM, mean fat cell mass = 0.750μg.
(c) shows adipose tissue from the upper thigh *before* weight reduction. Mean fat cell diameter (±s.d.) = 116.6±23.4μM, mean fat cell mass = 0.861μg.
(d) shows adipose tissue from the upper arm *after* weight reduction. Mean fat cell diameter (±s.d.) = 86.3±17.7μM, mean fat cell mass = 0.351μg.
(e) shows adipose tissue from the abdomen *after* weight reduction. Mean fat cell diameter (±s.d.) = 104.0±13.2μM, mean fat cell mass = 0.57μg.
(f) shows adipose tissue from the upper thigh *after* weight reduction.Mean fat cell diameter (±s.d.) = 94.9±15.1μM, mean fat cell mass = 0.45μg.
See 'Acknowledgements'

The relationship between adipose tissue cellularity and the natural history of obesity

The extra fat stored in the body of an obese individual is obviously stored in his fat cells, but the question which has been uppermost in the minds of researchers over the last 15 years is whether the extra fat is stored in existing fat cells, thus causing adipose cell hypertrophy or whether new fat cells are formed to accommodate it, thus leading to adipose cell hyperplasia. The other aspects which have received much attention are whether adipose cell hyperplasia can occur in response to external influences, and thus act as a trigger for obesity, and whether there are sensitive periods for the recruitment of new cells.

Despite the limitations of the methods for determining cell size and number, there is no doubt that individuals with the same amount of body fat can show considerable variation in mean fat cell size and therefore total fat cell number. In the early 1970s it was fashionable to relate fat cell number to the age of onset of obesity, and several publications reported that subjects with an early age of onset of obesity tended to be more hyperplastic than those whose obesity was adult-onset (Brook, Lloyd & Wolf, 1972; Salans, Cushman & Weismann, 1973). Reports such as these, taken together with convincing experiments involving the over-feeding of young animals, were over-interpreted and led to the widely reported 'fat cell hypothesis' which can be defined as follows: (1) overfeeding in early life causes the production of 'excess' fat cells, (2) the possession of 'excess' fat cells confers on that individual a predisposition to obesity.

Although the hypothesis did some good by placing emphasis on the prevention of overfeeding in early life, it possibly did an equal amount of harm because it led to the adoption of a 'fatalistic' approach to the treatment of individuals who had been obese since childhood.

More recently, several groups of workers have seriously questioned the original 'fat cell hypothesis' and have shown that the severity of obesity is a much more important determinant of total fat cell number than the age of onset of obesity (Ashwell, Priest & Bondoux, 1975; Hirsch & Batchelor, 1976). Thus it is now thought that a positive energy balance at any time of life will lead to the condition of obesity which is characterised either by large fat cells or by more fat cells, or by both.

The relationship between adipose tissue cellularity and the treatment of obesity
The second part of the 'fat cell hypothesis' of the early 1970s stated that the 'excess' fat cells would confer upon an individual a predisposition to obesity (see above). This view was founded on evidence that, in contrast to fat cell size which decreases, fat cell number remained constant when a group of individuals underwent weight reduction (Hirsch & Knittle, 1970; Björntorp & Sjöström, 1971). Re-examination of these publications shows that on average this seems to be true. However, Garrow (1978*a*) has pointed out that this statement is of the 'constancy fallacy' type and whereas there may be no general change in fat cell number in the group as a whole, there are certainly some members of the group who show large increases or decreases in fat cell number.

Perhaps the most important question to ask is 'Can the determination of adipose tissue cellularity give any clues to the prognosis for weight reduction?' If so, a simple, relatively painless biopsy would tell the clinician which of his patients would benefit from protracted, costly treatment.

Several groups have investigated the relationship between adipose tissue cellularity and weight loss. Studies of weight loss on a known energy intake have lasted only a few weeks; those lasting over a much longer timespan have been conducted as outpatient trials when it is impossible to achieve such a tight control of energy intake. An example of a short-term investigation is that of Ashwell, Durrant & Garrow (1978*b*); 33 women were studied in a research unit where food intake was strictly limited to 3.35 MJ (800 kcal) over a three-week inpatient period. A mean weight loss of nearly 5 kg was achieved and this was positively correlated with total fat cell number ($P<0.01$). However, when the severity of obesity was allowed for, the correlation of weight loss with fat cell number was not statistically significant. In fact, the best predictor of weight loss was resting metabolic rate which had a correlation coefficient of 0.73 ($P<0.001$) with weight loss.

The best study so far of the relationship between adipose tissue cellularity and long-term weight reduction is that of Krotkiewski *et al.* (1977). A group of 90 obese women on a standard outpatient diet of 4.60 MJ (1100 kcal) per day were divided into four groups on the basis of their adipose tissue cellularity ('borderline', 'hypertrophic', 'hyperplastic' and 'combined'). They were followed over a treatment period of up to two-and-a-half years – although most patients had been lost by 18 months. The 'hyperplastic' and 'combined' groups lost weight at a faster rate initially than the 'hypertrophic' group, but maintained a steady weight for shorter time and regained weight more quickly. 'Combined' and 'hyperplastic' groups invariably start off fatter and heavier than the other groups and this must be taken into account when assessing results; in this case, the rate of initial weight loss was higher and the duration of steady weight was shorter in the 'hyperplastic' compared with the 'hypertrophic' group, even when allowances were made for body fat. Krotkiewski *et al.* (1977) concluded that 'the long-term prognosis for weight reduction is worse for hypercellular forms of obesity than for the hypertrophic form. However, this does not mean that patients with hypercellular forms of obesity should not be treated at all since their spontaneous weight development might be lessened by repeated treatments.'

Future research in the role of adipose tissue in human obesity

The existence of fat cell precursors in human adipose tissue is now recognised (Van, Bayliss & Roncari, 1976). Although their identification has not been adequately confirmed, and the factors controlling their existence are not fully understood (Ashwell, 1978), they may provide the relationship between adipose tissue and the natural history and treatment of obesity.

Energy intake

The regulation of energy intake

The older studies of food intake in animals showed that many species can regulate their intake within very fine limits. When the energy density of stock diet was halved, rats ate double the weight of food and maintained body weight. Conversely on a high-energy-density diet rats reduced the weight of food eaten and did not gain weight (Adolph, 1947). Recently it has been shown that even rats can be fooled. High-fat diets (Schemmel, Mickelsen & Tolgay, 1969) and high-sucrose diets (Kanarak & Hirsch, 1977) can cause weight gain or increase in the proportion of body fat in some strains of animals. Animal models of dietary obesity have been described (Sclafani & Springer, 1976; Rolls & Rowe, 1977; Stock & Rothwell, 1978). Rats gain weight rapidly by overeating when they are fed snack, supermarket or cafeteria type foods similar to those consumed by humans.

Experiments on the regaulation of food intake in humans are less conclusive. Jordan (1975) has extensively studied intake of liquid-formula diet, either taken from a food-dispensing machine or fed intragastrically. Intake is maintained by either method independently, but when preloads are given intragastrically compensation is incomplete and slow. He suggests that this is evidence of sensory and oro-pharyngeal mechanisms for food intake regulation in humans. Jordan also concluded that volume was a more important factor than energy in determining food intake because a 1:9 dilution of the liquid diet caused a significant decrease in energy intake. However, the energy density of the diet was so low that it may have been beyond the capacity of some subjects to drink the quantity of fluid necessary for weight maintenance.

Spiegel (1973) gave normal-weight subjects preloads which were of constant volume but which varied in energy density. Intake of a milk formula preparation some time later was unrelated to the energy content of the preload and subjects did not show consistent compensation for meal size. In a further long-term study people were fed milk diet for four baseline days, followed by liquid in which energy density was halved for a further 1 - 2 weeks. According to their responses, the 15 subjects were classified as six regulators, six non-regulators and there were three who failed to increase their intake, but did not lose weight like the other non-regulators.

The only study to report good regulation in lean subjects was that of Campbell, Hashim & Van Itallie (1971). All five normal-weight male students adjusted promptly to changes in energy density of the liquid food. Changes in intake were in the right direction and were better than obese subjects but were not complete. Obese people using the same food-dispensing machine, decreased their intake and did not respond to changes in energy density. This could have been due either to motivation to lose weight or dislike of the liquid diet. It does not necessarily indicate a defect in food intake regulation in the obese.

Wooley (1971) gave liquid milk diets of disguised energy content to institutionalised, non-obese and obese patients for five baseline days. Low-energy-density milk formula was fed for the next five days and then followed by high-energy-density milk formula for the last five days. The subjects showed a partial adjustment of intake, drinking a greater volume of low-energy milk formula and a lower volume of high-energy milk formula, but the shifts in direction were insufficient to cause complete compensation. Energy intake was higher, 12.83MJ vs 8.03MJ (3066 kcal vs 1920 kcal) on the high-energy-density milk. The obese were no better or worse at regulation than non-obese subjects but the former did report more hunger.

The results of these studies show that individuals vary in their ability to regulate intake and that, although some obese people may be poor regulators, so too are a large proportion of normal-weight people.

Possible mechanisms for the regulation of food intake
Many physiological mechanisms for the regulation of food intake have been studied in animals (see Bray & Campfield, 1975*).

Neural. The earliest studies showed that lesions in the lateral and ventromedial hypothalamus caused aphagia and hyperphagia respectively. Electrical stimulation of these areas had the opposite effect, so they were called the feeding and satiety centres. Temperature may exert an effect on regulation by causing increased food intake in the cold and decreased food intake in the warm. Obesity in animals with lesions of the ventromedial hypothalamus can be prevented by vagotomy and a neural hormonal interaction is implied.

Recent studies of neural pathways have used staining techniques specific for different neurotransmitters. They show the location of the specific neural tracts and give evidence for the role of both catecholaminergic and serotinergic mechanisms in the neural control of feeding.

Hormonal. Obesity can be induced by injecting insulin whereas its metabolic counterpart, glucagon, has the opposite effect. Many other hormones have secondary effects on body weight or composition. Cushing's syndrome, which is due to excessive production of gluco-cortico steroids, is accompanied by obesity, whereas growth hormone therapy in rats increases lean body mass and decreases the proportion of fat. Gut hormones are secreted as food passes into the intestine and there is evidence that these may act on the satiety centres. Female reproductive hormones also affect body weight and hunger, but their role in energy intake regulation is not clear.

Peripheral. Short-term regulation of food intake is influenced directly by ingested food. Blood glucose levels have been shown to affect the activity of feeding centres of the hypothalamus and cause hunger in the fasted and satiety in the fed states. Free fatty acid levels in blood follow an opposite pattern to blood glucose and may be another signal. Amino acids have marked effects on food intake which is decreased both when essential amino acids are omitted or in excess, or when very-high-protein diets are fed.

Long-term regulation of energy stores has been implicated by several lipectomy studies which show that body fat tends to revert to its former level. Several workers have suggested that the amount of fat is signalled to the brain by a fat-soluble factor, but as none has been identified the concept remains hypothetical.

Do obese people have a defect in the regulation of energy intake?
Much research on human eating patterns is based upon the hypothesis that overweight people have a defect in regulation of food intake.

Stunkard (1959), by recording pressure change in a balloon attached to a stomach tube, showed that reported hunger was unrelated to movements of the stomach in the obese subjects. However these poor correlations were the result of a few patients with what he termed 'night eating syndrome' so it is not surprising that they did not report hunger during the day. In later studies (Stunkard & Fox,

**Many of these mechanisms are relevant to human feeding behaviour, but the invasive nature of some of the experimental techniques makes it difficult to test the contribution of such factors in the human situation.*

1971) gastric motility was shown to be poorly related to hunger in most normal subjects too.

Schachter (1968) extended this theory in a more general form and proposed that the eating behaviour of normal-weight subjects is related to their physiological or internal state but that obese people are influenced more by external stimuli such as food palatability, availability, prominence, time of day and social setting. For example, after eating roast-beef sandwiches non-obese subjects ate fewer biscuits at a later occasion, but obese people did not reduce their intake of biscuits.

Recent support for the internal-external theories has been shown by Pudel & Oetting (1977). In one experiment they gave women identical soups which had been labelled to indicate an energy content of 100-500 kcal. Satiety ratings were made immediately and one hour after a meal. They found that in obese subjects satiety was correlated with the false label when the discrepancy between labels was high. Normal-weight subjects were not so easily fooled as the obese.

In a second test they devised a sophisticated liquid-food-dispensing machine where the true feeding reservoir was hidden from the subject's view. The subject could only see the rate of emptying of a second reservoir whose emptying was independently controlled by the experimenter. In this way external influences on intake could be studied. They showed that normal weight people were better at maintaining constant intake despite changes in apparent intake, whereas obese people were more influenced by what they thought they had eaten. They also defined a group of people who were within 5 per cent of normal weight but had been overweight at some time previously. These 'latent obese' people showed responses similar to those of the obese subjects, showing that although they could maintain their weight they did it by exercising willpower rather than internal control. Although these test situations are somewhat artificial, Bruch (1973) has observed people who are unable to recognise internal signals of satiety. She questions the view that feeding is an innate response and emphasises the importance of early learning experiences in acquiring correct eating patterns. Emotional states can be mislearned, or become misassociated with hunger and feeding, if inappropriate conditioning occurs in infancy or childhood.

However, many experiments have failed to replicate the internal-external differences between obese and non obese subjects. Price & Grinker (1973) reported no significant difference between the number of crackers eaten in the preloaded and non-preloaded conditions for either obese or normal weight subjects. Wooley (1972) used drinks of either 0.84 or 2.51 MJ (200 or 600 kcal) each of which could be disguised as rich milk shakes or low energy liquid diet. Subjects believed both high and low-energy milk shakes to be higher in energy content than the high and low-energy liquid diet. On four consecutive days one of each of the preloads was given and 20 minutes later sandwiches were presented. The intake of sandwiches was unrelated to the *actual* energy content of the preloads in obese and non-obese people but was related more to *belief* about the energy content.

Wooley, Wooley & Dunham (1972) designed further tests where more time was allowed for the preloads to take effect and patients were encouraged to observe internal cues by reporting their hunger and satiety. Hunger was highly inversely related to patient guesses but not to actual energy content, showing again that cognitive belief rather than physiological signals were more influential for both groups.

Durrant & Mann (1977) have reported the only study to show that obese people *can* detect small differences in the energy content of food. During an eight-hour period on two consecutive days, energy intake was changed two-fold by a change in energy content of disguised food and patients were required to choose the day on which they were fed more; subjects guessed correctly 15 out of 19 times ($P<.05$) and hunger and appetite scores were inversely related to energy intake.

Palatability. Nisbett (1968) tested subjects' response to good and bad tasting ice-cream. Obese subjects and normal-weight subjects ate similar amounts of ice-cream rated poor in taste, but the obese ate more if they rated it good. Price & Grinker (1973) found similar results with biscuits. Cabanac & Duclaux (1970) described an effect called 'alliesthesia' where normal-weight people rated sweet solutions as less pleasant after a meal. Obese people reported no such effect.

Wooley, Wooley & Tennenbaum (1975) observed 2500 meal choices of obese or normal-weight subjects at a mediocre institutional cafeteria and a suburban cafeteria serving highly attractive, well-presented meals. The obese ate very slightly less at the plain, but significantly more at the fancy, cafeteria. Goldman, Jaffa & Schachter (1968) reported a tendency of obese college students to cancel refectory food and eat elsewhere. Therefore obese subjects appear to be more responsive to the palatability and sensory qualities of food than non-obese people.

Stress. It is difficult to manipulate stress in a controlled experimental situation but Rodin (1973) has described obese people as being more 'stimulus-bound' than normal-weight people. They are more responsive to prominent stimuli and are more easily distracted by disturbing pictures or tape recordings. Meyer & Pudel (1972) used monotonous irregular noises and insoluble puzzles on subjects whilst drinking liquid food. There was a tendency for the obese to eat more than the underweight or normal weight people in these stress conditions

Do obese people eat more than thin people?

Support for the view that not all overweight people are gluttons, came from the studies of Widdowson & McCance as long ago as 1936. They used the records of accurately weighed food intakes of 63 men and 63 women and found a two fold range of food intake within each group. Energy intake was not correlated with body weight expressed as a percentage of ideal weight. Similarly Durnin *et al.* (1974) made a cross sectional study over seven years on 611 adolescents. Food intake was measured over seven days and there was no significant difference between the energy intake of the thinnest and fattest boys, and the fattest girls ate significantly less (7.0 MJ/d) than the thinnest girls (9.23 MJ/d).

As long ago as 1900, Van Noorden described two types of obesity: exogenous (normal metabolism, high energy intake) or endogenous (pathogically diminished metabolism). These two extremes of a spectrum of causes of obesity have been described by other workers. Mayer made a similar distinction when he coined the terms 'regulatory' and 'metabolic' obesity. Clearly, some but not all obese people, find it difficult to restrain their food intake, just as the rats do when they are fed highly palatable food. But food intake is only one side of the energy balance equation. Maintaining food intake below sociably acceptable norms, or family pressures, may be a battle which the person with lower than average energy expenditure may not be able to sustain.

Energy expenditure

The total energy expenditure of any individual is composed of three parts: basal metabolism, thermogenesis, and physical activity. In this section, we will consider first the measurement of total energy expenditure and then see how the three separate components relate to the natural history of obesity.

Measurement of energy expenditure

The most accurate method of determining the total energy expenditure is to confine a subject in a thermostatically controlled chamber, a *direct calorimeter,* and to measure his total heat output over 24 hours or more. Unfortunately this method is very expensive and laborious and so energy expenditure is usually measured by the less accurate method of *indirect calorimetry,* ie measurement of oxygen consumption. Many types of apparatus have been designed for this purpose but most are uncomfortable, and none are suitable for measurements lasting for more than a few hours at the most. So, to measure the total energy expenditure by indirect calorimetry, the subject has to record all his activities on a special card, the energy cost of each of these must be determined, and the total computed by multiplying the time spent by the appropriate minute-energy cost. The limitations of this method have been reviewed by Durnin & Brockway (1959).

Another method for measuring the total expenditure involves the continuous monitoring of the heart rate and is based on the assumption that heart rate and energy expenditure are linearly related (Bradfield, 1971). Unfortunately there is some doubt about this relationship at lower levels of activity and it is unlikely that this method is any more accurate than the diary card method, although it is more socially acceptable. In fact, it is doubtful if either method is capable of measuring the daily energy expenditure of individuals with an accuracy of greater than ±10 per cent, so it may well be impossible to detect any small individual differences in total energy expenditure.

Basal metabolism

Basal metabolic rate (BMR) is defined as the energy expenditure of a subject under standardised conditions (ie after an overnight fast and while mentally and physically at rest in a thermoneutral environment). For most people, it is by far the largest component of the total energy expenditure. It is therefore important to know whether obese people have low BMRs, since this could go a long way toward explaining their obesity.

It is well established that BMR is affected by factors such as age, sex, and body size; and nomograms have been devised to predict energy expenditure accordingly. Table 4 shows the predicted BMRs of several hypothetical individuals and these have been increased and decreased by 10 per cent which is the accepted range of 'normal' variation. The table shows first that, on average, men have greater BMRs than women. Secondly, the range of BMRs is very large even for normal weight individuals (eg compare Mrs T.N. and Mrs S.N.). Thirdly, Table 4 shows that, although obese people should have *higher* BMRs than normal weight people as a result of their greater weight, this is not necessarily so if the obese individual has a BMR which is 10 per cent *less* than predicted and the normal weight individual has a BMR 10 per cent *greater* than predicted (compare Mrs A.N. and Mrs M.O.).

Table 4. Predicted basal metabolic rate (BMR) (±10%) for hypothetical men and women of different body size

Subject	Wt	Ht	Age	BMR (kcal/day)			BMR (mJ/day)		
	(kg)	(cm)	(yr)	Pred*	+10%	-10%	Pred*	+10%	-10%
Mr Small Normal (S.N.)	60	170	25	1650	1815	1485	6.91	7.60	6.22
Mr Average Normal (A.N.)	70	180	25	1850	2035	1665	7.75	8.53	6.98
Mr Tall Normal (T.N.)	80	190	25	2050	2255	1845	8.59	9.45	7.73
Mrs Small Normal (S.N.)	45	150	25	1180	1298	1062	4.94	5.44	4.45
Mrs Average Normal (A.N.)	55	160	25	1350	1485	1215	5.66	6.22	5.09
Mrs Tall Normal (T.N.)	65	170	25	1520	1672	1368	6.37	7.01	5.73
Mrs Moderately Obese (M.O.)	75	160	25	1550	1705	1395	6.49	7.14	5.85
Mrs Very Obese (V.O.)	110	160	25	1850	2035	1665	7.75	8.53	6.98

* BMR predicted from the nomogram of Boothby & Berkson (1933)

People with a tendency to obesity might be assumed to have BMRs which are consistently lower than the predicted value. However, although it has been reported that some obese people have low BMRs (Miller & Parsonage, 1975; James *et al.*, 1978; Griffiths & Payne, 1976) the majority of workers have reported the BMRs of obese people to be essentially normal or elevated (Grande, 1968).

Another important factor which affects the BMR is the level of energy intake. It has been shown in both normal weight (Taylor & Keys, 1950) and obese subjects (Bray, 1969; Apfelbaum, Bostsarron & Lacatis, 1971; Garrow, 1978*a*) that there is a marked fall in BMR during dietary restriction. Figure 4 shows the relationship of BMR to body weight in patients in our metabolic unit who were given a diet, supplying 3.35 MJ (800 kcal) daily for three weeks. In all patients BMR decreased over the three weeks, and in most cases the decrease was greater than that which would be predicted simply from the loss of weight. This adaptation could partly explain reports of low BMR in obese patients after prolonged dieting.

There is also some evidence that BMR increases in response to over-feeding (Garrow, 1978*b*) although the effect may depend on the extent and duration of overfeeding (Glick *et al.*, 1977) or on the type of diet, (Goldman *et al.*, 1975) or on the tendency of the individual to obesity (Stordy *et al.*, 1977).

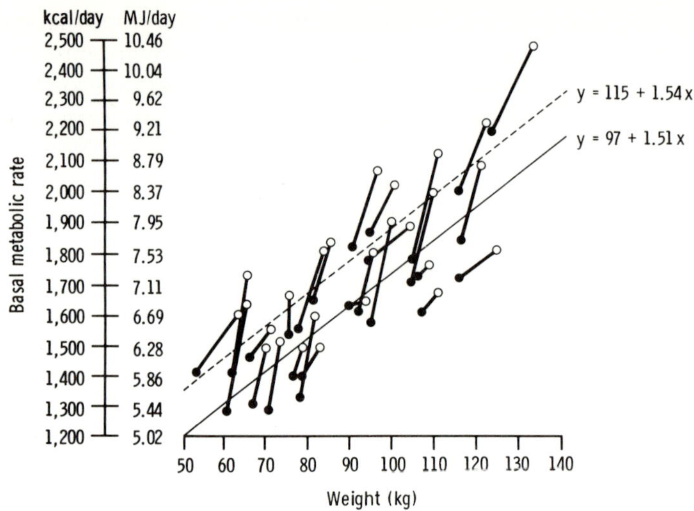

Fig. 4. Relationship of BMR to body weight in 26 patients in a metabolic ward who were given a 3.35MJ (800 kcal) diet daily for three weeks. The BMR against body weight of patients on admission to the research ward is shown as open symbols, and after three weeks on the diet as closed symbols. The relationship between BMR and body weight on admission is shown by the broken regression line (y=115 + 1.54x) and on discharge by the line y=97 + 1.51x. (This figure is based on data from Garrow & Warwick, 1978)

Thermogenesis

In recent years interest has revived in the phenomenon of thermogenesis, ie the increments to the BMR which occur in response to factors such as food, cold, drugs and hormones and which are unassociated with physical activity. Very little work has been done on obese:normal differences in response to drugs or hormones, so these will not be considered here. More work has been done on the effects of food and cold, and James & Trayhurn (1976) have formulated a hypothesis that obese subjects are limited in their ability to 'thermogen', and thereby have a reduced maintenance requirement. If this is so, they might also be limited in their ability to 'waste' excesses of intake when or if they should occur.

Response to food. This is the most important of the thermogenic factors and is generally thought to cause an extra expenditure equal to about 10 per cent of the ingested energy (Garrow, 1978*b*). Several studies have shown lower responses to food in obese than normal subjects (Pittet *et al.*, 1975; Kaplan & Leveille, 1976), and Stordy *et al.* (1977) found lower responses in overfed anorectics who had previously been obese than in those who had never been obese. On the other hand, some workers (Strang & McCluggage, 1931; Clough & Durnin, 1970; Bradfield & Jourdan, 1973) have failed to find lower responses in obese people which suggest either that some obese people can 'thermogen' normally, or that some normal people 'thermogen' abnormally.

Response to cold. Several workers have shown that fat subjects exposed to very low temperatures in near naked conditions show smaller increases in their metabolic rate than do normal weight subjects (Quaade, 1963; Wyndham, Williams &

Loots, 1968). Although these studies suggest an obese : normal difference in thermogenic ability, cold induced responses *per se* are probably unimportant in real life, since few people in their right mind expose themselves naked to the sort of low temperatures needed to produce them.

Quaade (1973) measured the response to cold in very lean, normal weight and obese subjects and found no difference between the obese and the normal although both groups responded less than the very lean. When he divided the obese group into those who admitted to overeating and those who did not, the over-eaters were found to respond *more* than the normals (and about the same as the very lean) but the non-overeaters showed no increase at all. This study illustrates the pitfalls in comparing 'thin' with 'fat' subjects, since there are obviously different 'types' in each group. Thus some of the confusion in the literature could be due to a failure to classify the 'type' of subjects studied.

Physical activity

Numerous studies have appeared attempting to relate obesity to physical inactivity and the reader is referred to Lutwak & Coulston (1975) or to Warwick (1978) for a review of the literature. Obese people are usually observed to be less active than normal weight people, but the literature is by no means conclusive on the subject. There is a wide range of activity between individuals in the same weight group and there are usually some obese who are more active than some normals. There is certainly no clear cut difference between obese and normal people in this respect and it is important to remember that the 'obese' are almost certainly not a homogenous group with respect to their level of activity. This may explain some of the discrepancies in the literature. Moreover, a low level of physical activity does not necessarily lead to a lower energy expenditure because the reduction might be offset by a weight related increase in energy cost.

In conclusion, there is clearly more energy expended for a given chore with added body mass, but there are tremendously wide individual variations both in the obese and in normal individuals. There may well be some obese individuals with low BMRs, others with a limited ability to 'thermogen', others with reduced activity, and others with some combination of these problems. Thus, there is not, and probably never will be, a simple, clear cut relationship between level of activity, energy expenditure and obesity.

Treatment of Obesity

General principles

Obesity is a result of a failure to match energy intake with energy expenditure, so energy stores are excessive. Treatment involves reversing the imbalance, so the energy stores (chiefly fat) return to normal proportions. However it is not a simple matter to reverse a long-standing error in energy balance, just as it is a difficult task to correct imbalances in the economy of a large company, or of a whole country. Many solutions are offered by different experts; however, there are certain general principles which would be agreed by virtually everyone with experience in this field, and it is useful to state these at first, so they do not become obscured in the later discussion of details.

The first question to be considered is: 'Would this person benefit from weight loss?' Depending on the definition used, about one third of the adult population of this country is overweight (see Introduction). However many of the people seeking advice on weight loss are not in fact overweight. About 1 per cent of girls in their late teens become preoccupied with thinness, and are alarmed by the normal physiological increase in body fat which occurs after puberty. In a severe form this condition – anorexia nervosa – may lead to emaciation and death. Anyone offering advice on weight loss needs to be vigilant that the potential patient is actually overweight, and is not seeking to be unduly thin. For this purpose the chart shown in Fig. 5 is helpful, since the lines indicate the

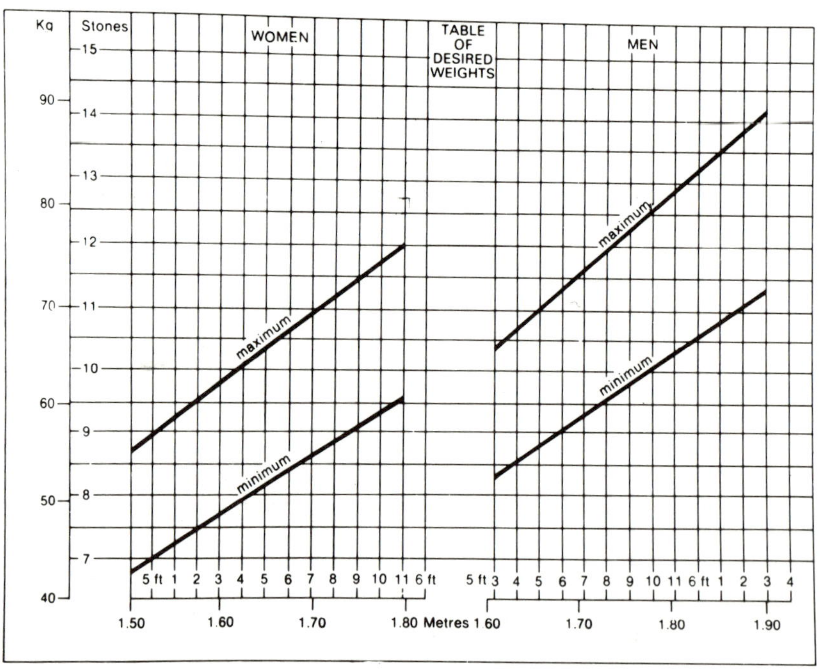

Fig. 5. Desirable weight range for men and women related to height (without shoes)

maximum and minimum 'desirable' weight for height in men and women. Here 'desirable' means associated with greatest life expectancy and good health, since the chart is constructed from the experience of the life insurance companies. Anyone outside the range, above or below, has a statistically worse expectation of life than a person of similar age and sex who is within the range, and the chances of good health and long life improve if an individual who was outside the range comes to lie within it (Dublin, 1963).

Decreasing energy intake

The mainstay of all treatment regimens for obesity is a low-energy diet. Since it is necessary to create a negative energy balance, this is most easily done by reducing the intake of energy from food so that it is less than the energy expenditure, and thus the excess energy stored in fat is burned to make good the energy deficit. The alternative (or additional) strategy of increasing energy expenditure is considered in the next section.

The most extreme form of reducing diet is total starvation. If no food is taken, and only acaloric fluids, then the whole energy requirements of the body must be met from the energy stores. This causes a very rapid weight loss, but it has serious drawbacks, so that it is not now generally used as a treatment for obesity. The clinical problems which arise with prolonged fasting are reviewed by Drenick (1976). Even with careful supplementation with vitamins and minerals, severe electrolyte disturbances may occur, and several patients have died with this treatment (Hermann & Iverson, 1968; Garnett *et al.*, 1969). The long-term results of starvation are also poor (Innes *et al.*, 1974). During the period of starvation weight is lost at about 3-4 kg per week, so in the series of 137 patients described by Drenick (1976) starvation for a period of 31-124 days caused a weight loss of 13-78 kg. However this weight tends to be regained more rapidly in patients who are starved than in those treated with a conventional low-energy diet (Maage & Morgensen, 1970). Probably this is because during total starvation much of the weight loss is lean tissue rather than fat, so at the end of treatment the patient has a relatively small lean body mass, and consequently a low basal metabolic rate (see p. 80).

Ideally a reducing diet should be acceptable to the patient, it should cause loss of fat with minimal loss of lean tissue, and it should be safe. No diet combines all these attributes perfectly, since it is obvious that the diet which was most acceptable to the patient was the one on which he or she became obese. It is unfortunate that the type of reducing diet which is most acceptable to patients is often one which causes rapid weight loss, such as starvation, but this is disappointing in the long run for reasons given above. Many attempts have been made to design 'protein-sparing modified fasts' which retain the advantages of rapid weight loss without the disadvantages of loss of lean tissue. If very low energy diets are to be used, say 250 kcal (1.05 MJ) per day, the diet needs to have a high protein content to reduce the loss of lean tissue. Flatt & Blackburn (1974) suggested that it was positively an advantage to exclude all carbohydrate from the diet, so the patient became ketotic, but Howard & Baird (1977) used a diet with 25 g of egg albumin as a protein source, and 40 g of carbohydrate which greatly reduced the ketosis. There is no general agreement that there is any benefit from ketosis: our own experience does not suggest that it protects the patient from the sensation of hunger.

A disadvantage of the 'protein-sparing fast' treatment is that the diet must be specially formulated to provide the necessary nutrients, so it is only suitable for use under skilled supervision, and cannot be achieved by modifying the diet which a housewife might normally be preparing for her family. If an energy value above 1000 kcal (4.18 MJ) per day is provided by the diet it becomes much less critical that the protein content should be high to preserve lean body mass, and if normal foods are used it is possible to supply the vitamin and mineral needs of the patient without using special supplements. However it requires some skill to devise a diet which is deficient in energy, but adequate in all other nutrients, and this is most easily done by reducing the intake of fried food, sugar and alcohol, since these items provide calories with little contribution to protein, mineral or vitamin intake. Advice along these lines is often misinterpreted: an obese patient may believe that provided certain 'fattening foods' are avoided anything else can be eaten in unlimited quantities, or else that provided enough salad vegetables (for example) are eaten, the requirements of a reducing diet are being fulfilled. It cannot be too strongly emphasised that the rate of weight loss is determined in the long run by the difference between energy intake and output, and since energy output varies greatly between individuals (see Table 4) so will the rate of weight loss on the same diet.

A device which is acceptable to many patients, safe, and often effective in causing weight loss is the low-carbohydrate diet (Yudkin, 1974). This diet is based on the principle that a person who is restricted in the amount of carbohydrate they can eat, will almost inevitably have a reduced energy intake, but will probably not be deficient in essential nutrients. Many general practitioners advise this diet (Craddock, 1973; Binnie, 1977), and it is probably a good first choice for moderately overweight people who have not tried dieting before. However it will not cause satisfactory weight loss in patients with a low total-energy expenditure, or in those who eat large quantities of foods which have little carbohydrate but a high energy content, like cheese.

Increasing energy expenditure

A person expends more energy when physically active than when at rest, so it is natural that patients think that if they lead a busy and tiring life they must have a high energy expenditure. Unfortunately this is not necessarily so. The values in Table 5 show the energy cost of walking at various speeds. To calculate the increase in energy expenditure of a man weighing 140 lb who walks, say, 4 miles each day at 4 miles per hour, it is necessary to estimate what his expenditure would have been had he not gone for this walk. If we suppose that at rest he used 1.2 kcal per minute, and while walking he uses 5.2 kcal per minute, then while he is walking he is using an extra 4 kcal per minute. During an hour he therefore uses an extra 240 kcal, which is roughly an increase of 10 per cent in daily energy expenditure. Since the variation between individuals in resting energy expenditure is at least 10 per cent a person who has a rather low resting metabolism and walks 4 miles per day will probably have about the same expenditure as someone with an average metabolism who takes no extra exercise.

Table 5. Energy expenditure (kcal/min) related to speed of walking (mph) and gross body weight (lb)(Passmore & Durnin, 1955).

	Weight						
Speed (mph)	80	100	120	140 (kcal/min)	160	180	200
2.0	1.9	2.2	2.6	2.9	3.2	3.5	3.8
2.5	2.3	2.7	3.1	3.5	3.8	4.2	4.5
3.0	2.7	3.1	3.6	4.0	4.4	4.8	5.3
3.5	3.1	3.6	4.2	4.6	5.0	5.4	6.1
4.0	3.5	4.1	4.7	5.2	5.8	6.4	7.0

Physical activity contributes to general fitness, but has a relatively small effect on energy expenditure. The complex literature on this subject has been reviewed in detail by Warwick (1978).

Apart from physical activity, the other means of increasing energy expenditure are discussed under the heading 'thermogenesis' (see p. 82). None of these is in practice very useful in the treatment of obesity. It is true that after a meal the metabolic rate increases, and thus there is an increase in energy expenditure, but this increase accounts for only about 10 per cent of the energy taken in the meal. In older textbooks the term 'specific dynamic action' is used to describe this increase, which was believed to be 'specific' for protein, but recent studies on human subjects have shown that the capacity of a meal to increase metabolism is related to its total energy content, and not to the amount of protein (Garrow & Hawes, 1972). It has even been claimed that certain foods, like hard boiled eggs, have a negative energy value, because the amount by which they increase metabolism is greater than their energy content, but this is untrue.

Exposure to severe cold will increase metabolism in the lightly clad subject, but this is a very unpleasant experience which no patient would choose as an alternative to dieting. There are several thermogenic drugs, of which the best-known is tri-iodothyronine, and with these it is possible to increase resting metabolism by about 30 per cent before side-effects become troublesome. However they are unsatisfactory for routine use, because they are potentially dangerous, and it requires very careful investigation to establish the correct dosage for individual patients. It is unlikely that a safe and useful thermogenic drug will be found for general use. Obese patients are handicapped by the fact that their exercise tolerance is limited by their extra weight, so they cannot maintain an increased energy expenditure without becoming very tired and breathless. The same problems arise if drugs are used to increase energy expenditure, but here the situation is more dangerous, since the energy expenditure cannot be suddenly decreased if, for example, the patient goes into heart failure. One of the great merits of exercise as a means of increasing metabolism is that it is so easily controlled, and if necessary stopped.

Alternative methods of treatment

Lipectomy. Patients seeking an effortless means of losing fat may be tempted to ask a surgeon to excise sheets of subcutaneous fat from the abdominal wall, buttocks or thighs. Unfortunately the result is never very satisfactory. An operation to cut away, say, 10 kg of fat involves undermining a large area of skin, and damaging its blood vessels and nerves, so during the healing process an unsightly scar forms. If the patient continues to lay down fat this piles up at the edge of the operation area, and makes it even less attractive. The effort involved in losing 10 kg of fat by following a normal reducing diet is not so great that anyone should resort to lipectomy, especially as the results of even the most skilled plastic surgeons are so poor both cosmetically and as a contribution to health.

Lipolytic agents. Many commercial slimming cures claim, or imply, that they cause fat to dissolve away without any direct action on energy intake or expenditure. This is impossible (see p. 83). Suppose that a drug or ointment were discovered which increased the rate at which the fat in adipose tissue was converted to fatty acid and released into the bloodstream. Fatty acids are insoluble in water, so to be transported safely in the blood they are carried on protein molecules, which would soon become saturated with fatty acid. At this stage no further fat could be mobilised until the carrier protein was unloaded, and this involves disposing of the fatty acid, either by burning it, or by depositing it back into fat somewhere else. If it is burned it replaces some other fuel, so on balance this enhanced lipolysis will have done nothing to reduce the fat stores of the body. On the contrary, there is cause for anxiety about any treatment which overloads the fat-transporting mechanism, since if circulating fatty acids are deposited as fat in, for example, the walls of the coronary arteries, this would do far more harm than leaving it in the adipose tissue. Any method which caused fat (as opposed to fatty acid) to leave the adipose tissue would be even more dangerous. Fat embolism is a hazard to people who have crush fractures of bone, since particles of fat may escape from the bone marrow and block up small vessels in the lung, thus causing pulmonary infarction. It is therefore just as well that 'cures' based on lipolysis do not work.

Decreased absorption
Medicines have been devised which coat the lining of the bowel to decrease absorption of food, or which decrease the efficiency of digestion. The problem about these treatments is that the bowel must be able to digest and absorb the essential nutrients, such as protein, vitamins and minerals, and the absorption of fat-soluble vitamins, and of minerals such as calcium, is dependent on the absorption of energy-providing nutrients such as fat. Thus it is unlikely that it will be possible to devise a treatment which selectively prevents absorption of energy from the diet, without also inhibiting the absorption of these essential nutrients.

The jejuno-ileal bypass operation was intended to decrease absorption of food, by short-circuiting all but 18 inches of small bowel. It does indeed decrease absorption, but the chief reason for weight loss after this operation is that the patient learns to eat less in order to avoid diarrhoea (Pilkington *et al.*, 1976). The malabsorption of vitamins and mineral after the operation requires careful management, and liver damage is an important complication.

Aids to decreased intake. Anorectic drugs such as diethylpropion, phentermine and fenfluramine decrease hunger, and at least in the short-term make it easier for the patient to tolerate a reducing diet. However there is no evidence that these drugs are very helpful in the long-term, since they tend to lose their effectiveness in a few weeks. Hunger is by no means the only reason for eating (see p. 77) so, even if hunger is abolished, patients do not necessarily find it easy to keep to a reducing diet. Factors such as social customs and the prominent display of food may make people eat when they are not hungry, so programmes of behaviour therapy have been devised to teach patients how to avoid stimuli which lead to eating. One of the best-known is that devised by Stuart (1967), which has since been modified by many other workers. Often patients can identify situations in which they eat for reasons other than hunger, and if they can arrange that these situations do not arise it will help them to reduce their food intake. Some patients try hypnosis, in the hope that this will enable them to reduce their food intake, but this does not seem to work as well as, for example, hypnosis for stopping smoking. Perhaps the reason is that it is more difficult to implant a hypnotic suggestion that the patient should eat less, than it is to cease smoking completely.

Less subtle, but more effective, methods of reducing food intake are by placing a mechanical obstruction in the way of eating. The simplest way of doing this is to wire the teeth together (Garrow, 1974), but this is not a satisfactory long-term solution. When the wires are removed after six to nine months the patient will probably have lost some 40 kg (6 stones) but usually most of the weight is regained in the next two years. A longer-term treatment is by gastric bypass (Mason & Ito, 1969), which reduces the size of the stomach, and hence the amount of food which can be taken at one meal. This operation compares favourably with jejunoileal bypass (Alden, 1977) since it produces comparable weight loss, but without the complications associated with malabsorption.

A practical plan for treatment of obesity

From the review above it will be evident that there is no single effective and acceptable treatment for obesity. Assuming that the patient is likely to benefit from weight loss (see General principles, above) the next step is to find out what treatment has been tried in the past, and why it failed. For purposes of this discussion let us first consider a person who is 10 kg (22 lb) above the maximum desirable weight for height (see Fig. 5), who has no physical disability arising from this, and who has made no serious attempt to lose weight before. For such a person a suitable rate of weight loss would be 2 lb (1 kg) per week for the first four weeks, and 1 lb (0.5 kg) a week thereafter. Thus it would take about 16 weeks to lose the excess weight, and this would be achieved with an average daily energy deficit of about 500 kcal (2.09 MJ) per day. The problem, therefore, is to find a diet acceptable to the patient, and which provides all the essential nutrients, but which provides about 500 kcal (2.09 MJ) per day less than the patient uses, so this deficit will be taken from the energy stores of the body. The reason for the more rapid loss of weight in the first four weeks is that the glycogen stores (see p. 70) are depleted at the start of a period on a reducing diet. It is not possible to estimate exactly the energy expenditure of the patient without calorimetry (see p. 80), but a diet supplying 1200 kcal (5.02 MJ) per day for a woman of average build, or 1500 kcal (6.27 MJ) for a man, should be about right. Attendance at a slimming club often helps patients in this category. If the required rate of weight loss is not attained, the diet should be adjusted accordingly.

If the patient has already had advice along the lines outlined above, and has failed to lose weight, the cause for this must be found. The most likely explanation is that the diet was not strictly observed, or too rapid a weight loss was expected. However, if neither of these explanations appears to apply the implication is that this patient has an unusually low metabolic rate. This could be verified by calorimetry, but usually this is not justified.

A more serious problem arises with a patient who is, say, 40 kg overweight, and who requires treatment such as an operation for gallstones or to replace a hip joint. Such patients are a bad surgical risk, and need to reduce weight before operation, but the rate of weight loss described above means that they would require 76 weeks to lose their excess weight, and this is a long time to wait for treatment of a painful condition. In these circumstances it is reasonable to aim for a more rapid weight loss by trying to achieve an energy deficit of about 1000 kcal (4.18 MJ) per day. In many patients this means an intake of about 800 kcal (3.34 MJ) per day, which is only achieved with very strict discipline. The problem is to find the diet in which the inconvenience to the patient is outweighed by the benefit from weight loss. The patient with painful joints or biliary colic stands to gain much from the operation, and is consequently motivated to accept a more rigorous diet. In these patients, in whom their obesity is presenting an immediate threat to health, it is indeed justified to carry out the appropriate investigations to determine their energy expenditure (Garrow, 1978*a*) if they fail to lose weight at the expected rate.

Conclusions

In this review we have tried to provide a summary of the current state of knowledge on certain aspects of obesity by assuming that obesity is a disorder of energy balance and examining in detail the three components of the energy balance equation. There are many other aspects of obesity which attract active research which we have not had the space to cover in this review. The reader who wishes to pursue the subject in greater detail would be well advised to refer to the three volumes of 'Recent advances in obesity research' (1974; 1978; 1981, in press) which contain the proceedings of the first three International Congresses of Obesity.

Acknowledgements — Tables 1 and 2 are adapted with permission of the publishers from similar tables in the DHSS/MRC Report 'Research on Obesity' (1976).

We are very grateful to Mr John Clark (Division of Electron Microscopy, Clinical Research Centre) for the photomicrographs (Fig. 3).

References

Adolph, E.F. (1947): *Am. J. Physiol.* **151**, 110-125.
Alden, J.F. (1977): *Archs Surg.* **112**, 799-806.
Apfelbaum, M., Botsarron, J. & Lacatis, D. (1971): *Am. J. Clin. Nutr.* **24**, 1405-1409.
Ashwell, M. (1975): *Hlth Educ. J.* **34**, 81.
Ashwell, M. (1978): *Int. J. Obesity* **2**, 69-72.
Ashwell, M.A., Priest, P. & Bondoux, M. (1975): In *Recent advances in obesity research*, **1**, ed A.N. Howard, p. 74. London: Newman.
Ashwell, M., Chinn, S., Stalley, S. & Garrow, J.S. (1978*a*): *Int. J. Obesity* **2**, 289-302.
Ashwell, M., Durrant, M. & Garrow, J.S. (1978*b*): *Int. J. Obesity* **2**, 449-456.
Baird, I.M., Silverstone, J.T., Grimshaw, J.J. & Ashwell, M. (1974): *Practitioner* **212**, 706.
Binnie, C.C. (1977): *J. Roy. Coll. Gen. Pract.* **27**, 492-495.
Björntorp, P. & Sjöström, L. (1971): *Metab.* **20**, 703.
Björntorp, P. (1978): In *Recent advances in obesity research. 2*, ed G.A. Bray, pp. 153-168. London: Newman.
Boothby, W.M. &Berkson, J. (1933 in 1975): In *Obesity in perspective*, ed G.A. Bray, Appendix IV, Table 7. Washington DC: Govt. Ptg. Off.
Bradfield, R.B. (1971): *Am. J. Clin. Nutr.* **24**, 1148-1154.
Bradfield, R.B. & Jourdan, M.H. (1973): *Lancet* **2**, 640-643.
Bray, G. (1969): *Lancet* **2**, 397-398.

Bray, G.A. & Campfield, L.A. (1975): *Metab.* **24**, 99-117.
Brillat-Savarin, J.A. (1889): *The physiology of taste,* Trans. R.E. Anderson. London: Chatto and Windus.
Brook, C.G.D., Lloyd, J.K. & Wolf, O.H. (1972): *Br. Med. J.* **2**, 25.
Bruch, H. (1973): *Eating disorders.* London: Routledge & Kegan Paul.
Cabanac, M. & Duclaux, R. (1970): *Science* **168**, 496-497.
Campbell, R., Hashim, S.A. & Van Itallie, T.B. (1971): *New Engl. J. Med.* **285**, 1402-1407.
Chicago Society of Actuaries (1959): *Build and blood pressure study.*
Clough, D.P. & Durnin, J.V.G.A. (1970): *J. Physiol. (Lond.)* **207**, 89P.
Craddock, D. (1973): In *Obesity and its management,* 2nd edn. London: Churchill-Livingstone.
Department of Health & Social Security/Medical Research Council (1976): *Research on obesity.* London: HMSO.
Drenick, E.J. (1975): In *Obesity in perspective,* ed G.A. Bray, pp. 341-360. Washington DC: US Govt. Ptg. Off.
Dublin, L.I. (1953): *New Engl. J. Med.* **248**, 971-974.
Durnin, J.V.G.A. & Brockway, J.M. (1959): *Br. J. Nutr.* **13**, 41-53.
Durnin, J.V.G.A., Lonergan, M.E., Good, J. & Ewan, A. (1974): *Br. J. Nutr.* **32**, 169-179.
Durrant, M.L. & Mann, S. (1977): *Proc. Nutr. Soc.* **36**, 113A.
Flatt, J.P. & Blackburn, G.L. (1974): *Am. J. Clin. Nutr.* **27**, 175-187.
Garnett, E.S., Barnard, D.L., Ford, J., Goodbody, R.A. & Woodhouse, M.A. (1969): *Lancet* **1**, 914-916.
Garrow, J.S. (1974): *Proc. Nut. Soc.* **33**, 29A.
Garrow, J.S. (1978*a*): *Energy balance and obesity in man,* 2nd edn. Amsterdam: North-Holland.
Garrow, J.S. (1978*b*): In *Recent advances in obesity research, 2.* ed G.A. Bray, p. 200. London: Newman.
Garrow, J.S. & Hawes, S.F. (1972): *Br. J. Nutr.* **27**, 211-219.
Garrow, J.S. & Warwick, P.M. (1978): In *Diet of man: needs and wants,* ed J. Yudkin, pp. 127-144. London: Applied Science.
Glick, Z., Schvartz, Z.E., Magazanik, A. & Modan, M. (1977): *Am. J. Clin. Nutr.* **30**, 1026-1035.
Goldman, R., Jaffe, M. & Schachter, S. (1968): *J. Person. Soc. Psychol.* **10**, 117.
Goldman, R., Haisman, M., Bynum, G., Horton, E.S. & Sims, E.A.H. (1975): In *Obesity in perspective,* ed G.A. Bray, pp. 165-186. Washington DC: US Govt. Ptg. Off.
Grande, F. (1968): *Am. J. Clin. Nutr.* **21**, 305-314.
Griffiths, M. & Payne, P.R. (1976): *Nature* **260**, 698-700.
Gurr, M.I. & Kirtland, J. (1978): *Int. J. Obesity* **2**, 401-427.
Hermann, L.S. & Iverson, M. (1968): *Lancet* **2**, 217.
Hirsch, J. & Batchelor, B. (1976): *Clins Endocrin. Metab.* **5**, 299.
Hirsch, J. & Knittle, J.L. (1970): *Fed. Proc.* **29**, 1516.
Howard, A. & McLean Baird, I. (1977): *Int. J. Obesity* **1**, 63-78.
Innes, J.A., Campbell, I.W., Campbell, C.J., Needle, A.L. & Munro, J.F. (1974): *Br. Med. J.* **2**, 356.
James, W.P.T. & Trayhurn, P. (1976): *Lancet* **2**, 770-773.
James, W.P.T., Davies, H.L., Dauncy, M.J. & Bailes, J. (1978): *Int. J. Obesity* **2**, 394-395.
Jordan, H.A. (1975): In *Obesity in perspective,* ed G.A. Bray, pp. 35-47. US Govt. Ptg. Off.
Kanarek, R.B. & Hirsch, E. (1977): *Fed. Proc.* **36**, 154-158.
Kaplan, M.L. & Leveille, G.A. (1976): *Am. J. Clin. Nutr.* **29**, 1108-1113.
Khosla, T. & Lowe, C.R. (1968): *Lancet* **1**, 742.
Krotkiewski, M., Sjöström, L., Björntorp, P., Carlgren, G., Garrellick, G. & Smith, U. (1977): *Int. J. Obesity* **1**, 395.
Lutwak, L. & Coulston, A. (1975): In *Obesity in perspective,* ed G.A. Bray, pp. 393-396. Washington DC: US. Govt. Ptg. Off.
Maage, H. & Morgensen, E.F. (1970): *Dan. Med. Bull.* **17**, 206-209.
Mason, E.E. & Ito, C. (1969): *Ann. Surg.* **170**, 329-336.

Meyer, J.E. & Pudel, V. (1972): *J. Psychosom. Res.* **16**, 305-308.
Miller, D.S. & Parsonage, S. (1975): *Lancet* **1**, 773-775.
Montegriffo, A.N. (1971): *Postgrad. Med. J.* **47**, suppl. 418.
Nisbett, R.E. (1968): *J. Personality Soc. Psychol.* **10**, 107-116.
Passmore, R. & Durnin, J.V.G.A. (1955): *Physiol. Rev.* **35**, 801-840.
Pilkington, T.R.E., Gazet, J-C., Ang, L., Kalucy, R.S., Crisp, A.H. & Day, S. (1976): *Br. Med. J.* **1**, 1504-1505.
Pittet, Ph., Chappuis, Ph., Acheson, K., Techtermann, F. de & Jequier, E. (1976): *Br. J. Nutr.* **35**, 281-292.
Price, J.M. & Grinker, J. (1973): *J. Comp. Physiol. Psychol.* **85**, 265-271.
Pudel, V.E. & Oetting, M. (1977): *Int. J. Obesity* **1**, 369-386.
Quaade, F. (1963): *Lancet* **2**, 429-432.
Quaade, F. (1973): In *Energy balance in man,* ed M. Apfelbaum, pp. 135-140. Paris: Masson.
Recent advances in obesity research, 1. (1974): ed A.N. Howard, London: Newman.
Recent advances in obesity research, 2. (1978): ed G.A. Bray. London: Newman.
Recent advances in obesity research, 3. (1981): ed A.N. Howard. London: Libbey.
Richardson, A.N. & Pincherle, A.N. (1969): *Br. J. Prev. Soc. Med.* **23**, 267.
Rodin, J. (1973): *J. Comp. Physiol. Psychol.* **83**, 68-75.
Rolls, B.J. & Rowe, E.A. (1977): *J. Physiol.* **273**, 2P.
Salans, L.B., Cushman, S.W. & Weismann, R.E. (1973): *J. Clin. Invest.* **52**, 929.
Schachter, S. (1968): *Science* **161**, 751-756.
Schemmel, R., Mickelsen, O. & Tolgay, Z. (1969): *Am. J. Physiol.* **216**, 373-379.
Sclafani, A. & Springer, D. (1976): *Physiol. Behav.* **17**, 461-471.
Spiegel, T.A. (1973): *J. Comp. Physiol. Psychol.* **84**, 24-37.
Stock, M. & Rothwell, N. (1978): In *Animal models of obesity,* ed M.F.W. Festing. London: McMillan.
Stordy, B.J., Marks, V., Kalucy, R.S. & Crisp, A.H. (1977): *Am. J. Clin. Nutr.* **30**, 138-146.
Strang, S.M. & McCluggage, H.B. (1931): *Am. J. Med. Sci.* **182**, 49.
Stuart, R.B. (1967): *Behav. Res. Ther.* **5**, 357-365.
Stunkard, A. (1959): *Psychosom. Med.* **21**, 281-289.
Stunkard, A.J. & Fox, S. (1971): *Psychosom. Med.* **33**, 123-134.
Taylor, H.L. & Keys, A. (1950): *Science* **112**, 215-218.
Van, R.L.R., Bayliss, C.E. & Roncari, D.A.K. (1976): *J. Clin. Invest.* **58**, 699.
von Noorden, C. (1900): *Die Fettsucht.* Wien: Hoelder.
Warwick, P.M. (1978): The influence of Physical Activity on energy expenditure in man, and its role in the treatment of obesity. PhD These, University of London.
Widdowson, E.M. & McCance, R.A. (1936): *J. Hyg.* (Lond.) **36**, 269-309.
Wooley, O.W. (1971): *Psychosom. Med.* **33**, 436-444.
Wooley, S.C. (1972): *Psychosom. Med.* **34**, 62-68.
Wooley, O.W., Wooley, S.C. & Dunham, R.B. (1972): *J. Comp. Physiol. Psychol.* **80**, 250-258.
Wooley, S.C., Wooley, O.W. & Tennenbaum, O. (1975): In *Obesity: its pathogenesis and management,* ed T. Silverstone, pp. 101-102. Lancaster: Medical & Technical Publishing.
Wyndham, C.H., Williams, C.G. & Loots, H. (1968): *J. Appl. Physiol.* **24**, 282-287.
Yudkin, J. (1974): In *Obesity,* ed W.L. Burland, P.D. Samuel & J. Yudkin, pp. 271-280. Edinburgh: Churchill-Livingstone.

8

Diet and coronary heart disease

A.N. Howard.

Introduction

Coronary heart disease is now the major cause of death in many parts of the developed world. In England and Wales over 150 000 (30 per cent total) died from the disease in 1976 (Office of Population Censuses and Surveys, 1978). A number of facts are clearly established. The incidence of the disease varies greatly between one country and another. For example, Finland has 16 times more deaths per capita than Japan (Keys, 1970). It is a disease which has increased to epidemic proportions. Thus in England and Wales there was a two-fold increase in death rate from 1950-1970, and an annual increase has been evident since the beginning of the century (DHSS, 1974).

Because countries differ in the type of food they eat, and food consumption has changed both qualitatively and quantitatively since the beginning of the century, it is assumed that faulty nutrition is an important factor in the disease. There was a sharp fall in death rate from cardiovascular diseases during the 1939-1945 war in many European countries, especially in Scandinavia (Malmros, 1950). This was accompanied by a decrease in the consumption of many food-stuffs. After the war in Germany, with the greater availability of food, there was a massive increase in mortality from coronary heart disease (Schettler, 1950).

Epidemiological results can only give clues and provide hypotheses to be tested experimentally. Whilst there can be few nutritionists who would not agree that diet is implicated in the aetiology of coronary heart disease, the subject is one of great controversy. It is possible to show that most of the nutrients we eat, whether fat, protein, carbohydrate, vitamins or minerals, have changed either in consumption or quality over the years. Thus there can be as many hypotheses as nutrients in the diet.

Whilst nutrition may be a major factor, it certainly is not the only one. Age, sex, smoking habits, blood pressure, the amount of exercise taken and the presence of other conditions, such as obesity and diabetes, are of equal or often of greater importance. It is important to consider the interaction of these 'risk factors' with dietary factors (Lewis, 1978).

The majority of investigators believe that any effect of nutrition on coronary heart disease lies in changes in serum lipids and lipoproteins. Others feel that the problem is related to factors such as injury to the walls of the coronary arteries or the initiation and promotion of thrombosis therein.

The object of the present review is to present the facts as currently established, and particularly to draw attention to the experimental data to support the hypotheses.

Risk factors for coronary heart disease

1. Serum lipid and lipoproteins

Our knowledge of lipid metabolism has expanded enormously during the last 20 years, much of this being due to advances in separation techniques – electrophoresis, ultracentrifugation, nephelometry, thin-layer and gas chromatography. Cholesterol and triglycerides circulate in the blood as complex lipoproteins and these have been classified according to their separation by electrophoresis or ultracentrifugation (Fig. 1) into high density (HDL), low density (LDL), very low density (VLDL) and chylomicrons. As the particles increase in size they contain relatively more triglyceride and less cholesterol.

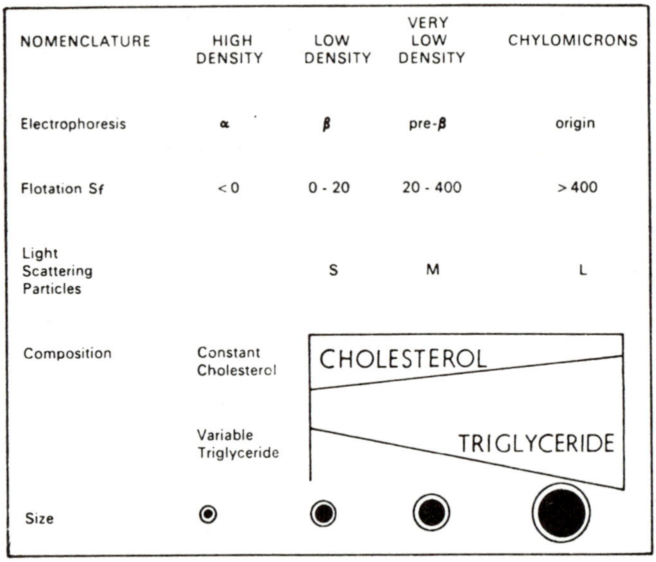

NOMENCLATURE	HIGH DENSITY	LOW DENSITY	VERY LOW DENSITY	CHYLOMICRONS
Electrophoresis	α	β	pre-β	origin
Flotation Sf	<0	0 - 20	20 - 400	>400
Light Scattering Particles		S	M	L
Composition	Constant Cholesterol Variable Triglyceride	CHOLESTEROL		TRIGLYCERIDE
Size				

Fig. 1. Nomenclature, composition and size of serum lipoproteins

The evidence that elevated serum lipids are one of the factors involved in coronary heart disease is very impressive. One of the most important studies (Kannel *et al.*, 1971) is that carried out in Framingham, Massachusetts (Fig. 2).

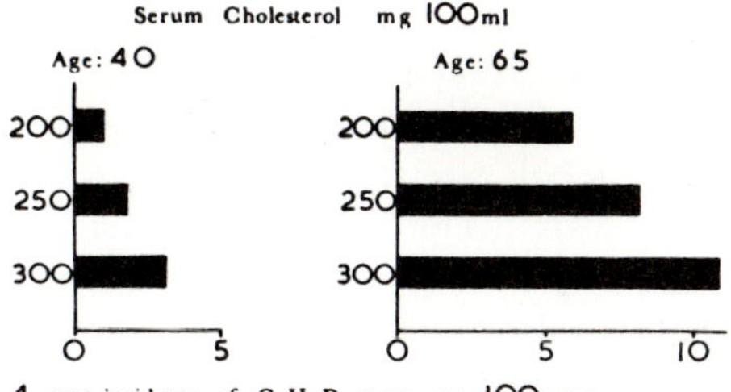

Fig. 2. Incidence of coronary heart disease at ages 40 and 65 in Framingham study (Dayton, 1972)

More than 5000 men and women aged 30-62 were studied for over 12 years in a prospective study. A clear-cut linear relationship between serum cholesterol and new coronary events was established. Thus, the chance of a man of forty developing coronary heart disease with a serum cholesterol of 300 mg/100 ml is three times greater than one with 200 mg/100 ml. Other prospective studies carried out at 20 centres throughout the world confirmed this result (Truswell, 1978).

The Framingham and other studies found that cigarette-smoking and high blood pressure were also risk factors. Moreover, the risk factors were independent and multiplicative. It is noteworthy that the Japanese who smoke as many cigarettes as Westerners and who develop high blood pressure, but have low serum cholesterol, rarely develop coronary heart disease (Keys, 1970). Thus it seems likely that some other risk factors may not operate in populations with low serum cholesterol.

The significance of triglycerides which occur chiefly in VLDL has been obscure until quite recently because of the lack of a clear-cut prospective study. However, Carlson & Bottinger (1972), in a nine-year follow up of over 3000 men in Stockholm, showed that coronary heart disease increased linearly with increasing fasting concentrations of plasma triglycerides, and that the risk was independent of plasma cholesterol. A combined elevation of these two plasma lipids carried the highest risk (Table 1). However, in eight other prospective studies, serum triglycerides were not found to be an independent predictor of coronary heart disease (Truswell, 1978). One view is that elevated triglycerides must be a secondary phenomenon related indirectly with other risk factors such as high cholesterol, diabetes, obesity, lack of exercise, mental stress and lower HDL.

Table 1. Risk of developing coronary heart disease in relation to serum cholesterol and triglycerides (Carlson & Bottinger, 1972)

	Group			
Serum	1	2	3	4
Cholesterol (>280mg/100ml)	Normal	Raised	Normal	Raised
Triglycerides (>170mg/100ml)	Normal	Normal	Raised	Raised
Rate CHD/10^3/year	7.3	15.6	26.8	31.3

For many years HDL was largely ignored, since only the other lipoproteins appeared to be incriminated in coronary heart disease. Recent evidence suggests that HDL may be of equal importance, but from a quite different aspect (Miller & Miller, 1975). A *reduction* of plasma HDL may accelerate the development of atherosclerosis and an increased level may be protective. The strongest of the experimental data to support this view is that the total body cholesterol pool increases with decreasing plasma HDL but is unrelated to plasma cholesterol or other lipoproteins.

Other evidence, mainly from *in-vitro* experiments, demonstrates that HDL facilitates the uptake of cholesterol from the peripheral tissues and its transport to the liver for catabolism and excretion. Plasma HDL is reduced in several conditions associated with an increased risk for coronary heart disease, namely cigarette-smoking, hypercholesterolaemia, hypertriglyceridaemia, male sex, obesity and diabetes mellitus. Patients with existing clinical coronary heart disease have lower levels of HDL than the normal population. There have been many prospective studies and the following is fairly typical.

In a study in Tromsø, Norway, over 6000 men aged 20-49 were examined for a number of risk factors (Miller *et al.*, 1977). Plasma from 17 patients with CHD was compared with a similar number of controls matched for plasma cholesterol, triglyceride concentration, systolic and diastolic blood pressures, relative body weight and cigarette consumption. The major difference between the two groups was in plasma HDL cholesterol concentration which averaged 35 per cent lower in CHD cases than in the controls. This difference applied not only to those cases who had already suffered a myocardial infarction before the start of the survey but also to those who were previously clinically healthy and then developed CHD. Although the other lipoprotein (LDL + VLDL) cholesterols were also positively correlated, HDL cholesterol made a three-fold greater prediction.

Probably one of the most convincing arguments in favour of the hypothesis is that it explains why women are protected from coronary heart disease since women have about 20 per cent more HDL-cholesterol than men. On the other hand, people with Tangier's disease, who have a virtual absence of HDL in their serum, do not suffer from coronary heart disease any more than the rest of the population (Assman & Schaefer, 1978). So the case for HDL-cholesterol is not cast iron.

2. Obesity

The death rate of obese people is higher than that of people of the same age who are not obese and this earlier mortality is in part due to death from coronary heart disease (Baird & Howard, 1969; Howard, 1975; Bray, 1978). Obesity is associated with physical underactivity, high blood pressure and diabetes mellitus, each of which is considered to be an important risk factor for coronary heart disease. Studies suggest that, in the absence of associated factors, obesity alone may not add much to the total risk. Obese people often have high serum triglycerides which return to normal after weight reduction, but there is only a weak association between obesity and serum cholesterol (Pelkonen *et al.*, 1977). In other words, an obese person who has normal serum lipids, blood pressure, and glucose tolerance and is physically active may have no greater risk of developing coronary heart disease than a normal-weight individual.

Specific nutrients and coronary heart disease

1. Dietary cholesterol

For over 50 years the relationship between diet and serum cholesterol has been established in animals. This stems from the classic work of Anitschkow who fed a diet of meat and fat to rabbits and produced arterial lesions in the aorta and coronary arteries (Anitschkow, 1933). He concluded that the causative factor was dietary cholesterol, since feeding pure cholesterol gave the same result. Later work with other species (eg rat, dog) showed that dietary cholesterol alone was insufficient, and that it was necessary to make the animals hypothyroid (using thiouracil) or to interfere with cholesterol metabolism by feeding cholic acid, so as to produce an intense hypercholesterolaemia (Howard & Gresham, 1968).

Application of these results to man soon proved a failure. Cholesterol feeding, even in massive doses, failed to affect serum cholesterol levels (Messinger, Poroswiska & Steele, 1950). The reasons put forward to explain this difference were numerous. In man, there is a limitation on the amount of cholesterol which can be absorbed. Furthermore, any dietary cholesterol absorbed forms part of the whole body pool so that the synthesis of cholesterol by the liver and other tissues is suppressed by a feed-back mechanism.

Nevertheless, dietary cholesterol has a small but definite influence on serum cholesterol. Up to an intake of 600 mg/day there is a linear relationship but the effect then reaches a plateau (Connor, Hodges & Bleiler, 1961). This may explain why investigators obtain such divergent results. Keys estimates that one egg (about 200 mg cholesterol) increases serum cholesterol by 5 to 6 mg/100 ml (Keys, 1967). However, there is a very wide individual response. Mistry *et al.* (1976) gave 14 normal subjects 750 mg cholesterol/day as egg yolk and obtained changes of -5 to +20 per cent in serum cholesterol. In another study, ten eggs gave rises of three to 57 per cent (Dam *et al.*, 1970). In a study in Missouri, one additional egg added to the diet/day had no effect (Porter *et al.*, 1977).

To summarise, the effect of changing the cholesterol content of the diet depends on the person's current intake. If it is in the region of 500-750 mg/day, any further quantities of cholesterol may have only a small additional effect. However, reducing cholesterol intake below this amount may achieve a considerable beneficial change in serum cholesterol.

The absorption of cholesterols also depends on other constituents in the diet. Dietary triglycerides increase cholesterol absorption and plant sterols, particularly β-sitosterol, inhibit (Kritchevsky, 1958). The latter is not absorbed itself and is thought to form a complex with cholesterol. Although β-sitosterol is used pharmaceutically as an agent to reduce serum cholesterol, large amounts have to be given (circa 15 g/day) and the quantities present in food are not sufficient to play a major role in cholesterol metabolism.

2. Dietary triglycerides

(i) Development of the dietary fat hypothesis

One of the earliest experiments which drew attention to the importance of dietary triglycerides was reported in 1950 by Ancel Keys & his colleagues, using the rice-fruit diet. This regime, consisting of only rice and fruit, was used extensively in the treatment of high blood pressure because of its very-low-sodium content. Patients on this diet have an abnormally low serum-cholesterol level, often 50 per cent below the pre-treatment value. Addition of a vegetable fat margarine, containing no cholesterol, returned the serum cholesterol to the original level. This isolated observation provoked the extensive examination of the effect of dietary triglycerides, as distinct from cholesterol, on serum cholesterol, and the incidence of coronary heart disease. The studies can be divided into two categories, epidemiological and experimental.

Following up his initial experimental observation, Keys was able to show that in countries where the percentage of calories consumed as fat was about 40 per cent, severe atherosclerosis was common, and serum cholesterol was high. In populations eating little fat, such as the African Bantu and the Japanese, the disease was rare, and serum cholesterol was low (Keys, 1970). Whilst these observations might be explained on genetic grounds, it was found that environment was more important. Thus, Japanese who have emigrated and live an American style life in Hawaii and California, have a higher incidence of the disease than those who remain behind in Japan (Worth *et al.,* 1975). The differences in fat intake run parallel. Further epidemiological studies showed that there was a greater statistical correlation with animal (saturated) fat than vegetable fat (Fig. 3).

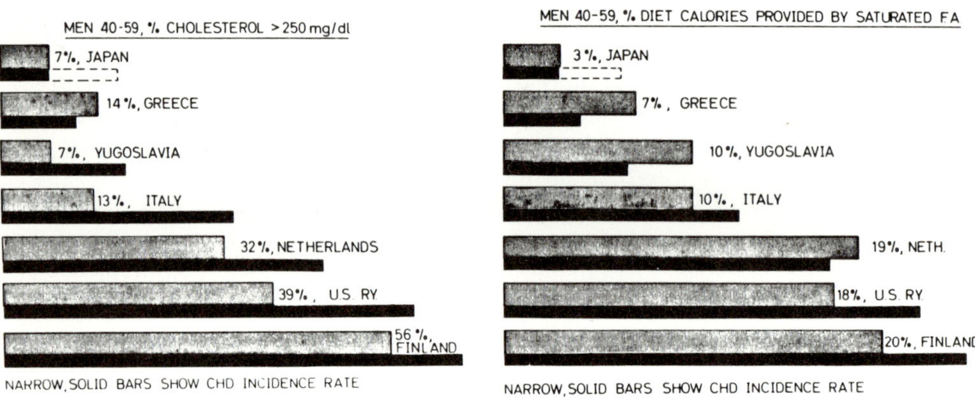

Fig. 3. Effect of serum cholesterol (left) and percentage of total dietary energy (right) provided by saturated fatty acids in relation to the incidence rate of coronary heart disease. (Incidents /10 000. Scale for Finland = 198) (Keys, 1970)

To give an example of a specific study, Bronte-Stewart, Keys & Brock (1955) studied the Bantu and Europeans in S. Africa. Extensive coronary heart disease is a rarity in the Bantu but very common in the European stock. The mean serum cholesterol of the two races was 166 mg/100 ml and 234 mg/100 ml and fat consumption 17 per cent and 37 per cent of total energy intake, respectively.

These epidemiological observations stimulated a study of experimental effects of feeding different fats in man. It was quickly found that not all fats behave the same. Animal fats such as butter, beef-dripping or tallow led to a prompt rise in serum cholesterol, whilst vegetable oils such as corn, sunflower and peanut, lowered them (Bronte-Stewart, 1958). Changes could be seen in 48 hours and usually reached a maximum in two to three weeks (Fig. 4). When the above-mentioned oils were hydrogenated their ability to decrease serum cholesterol was lost. The difference was not merely one of animal or vegetable origin, but of

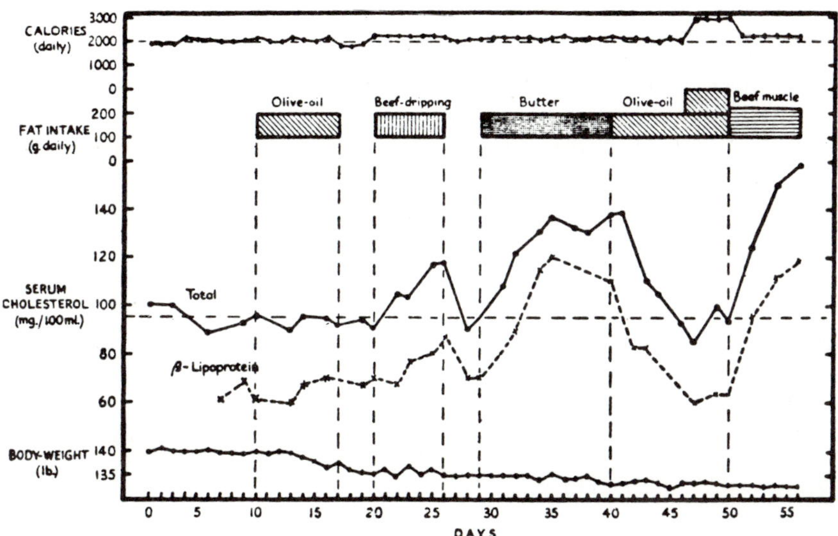

Fig. 4. Effects of different fats on serum cholesterol in a male Bantu (Bronte-Stewart, 1958)

saturation of the fatty acids. Thus, cocoanut and palm oil which contain chiefly saturated fatty acids, raise serum cholesterol, whereas fish oils which are highly unsaturated, lower it. Keys, Anderson & Grande (1965) after a very extensive study of the parameters involved, devised the following equation:

$$\Delta \text{ cholesterol} = 1.3 \quad (2\,\Delta\, S - \Delta\, P) + 1.5\ \Delta\, Z$$

where Δ cholesterol is the average change in serum cholesterol (mg/100 ml) and S and P are percentages of total calories from triglycerides of saturated and polyunsaturated fats respectively and Z is the square root of the dietary cholesterol expressed as mg/1000 kcal diet. Fatty acids which are mono-unsaturated – as for instance oleic acid, the main constituent of olive oil – have no effect.

The changes in serum cholesterol were due to low-density (β) lipoprotein and not the high-density (α) lipoprotein (Bronte-Stewart, 1958). Differences in energy, protein or vitamin intake did not appear to influence the response. Also it should be noted that polyunsaturated oils can neutralise the effect of saturated fat when fed simultaneously. Not all saturated fatty acids have an effect but only those which contain 12 to 14 carbon atoms. Stearic acid (18 carbons) is inactive, but this is usually a minor constituent of animal fat (Keys *et al.*, 1965).

To summarise, the dietary-fat hypothesis states that the level of serum cholesterol in man is related to the fatty-acid composition of the dietary triglycerides and to a lesser extent the cholesterol intake, and that these changes can influence the incidence and extent of coronary heart disease.

(ii) Paradoxical results
Almost all the experimental studies carried out in man have been concerned with the addition of isolated triglycerides to the diet. It has always been tacitly assumed that the consumption of foods containing these fats would have a similar effect. Such is not the case. Whole milk contains 50 per cent calories as butter fat, and drunk in large quantities should theoretically increase serum cholesterol. However, the consumption of two litres milk daily for two weeks causes a decrease in serum cholesterol of 5 per cent, whereas the equivalent quantity of butter contained in the milk produces a 17 per cent increase (Table 2) (Howard & Marks, 1977). These data suggest that milk may contain a factor which antagonises the cholesterol-raising properties of butter (Howard, 1977).

Table 2. Effect of milk products on serum cholesterol in normal people

Milk product	Dose/ day	No.	Serum cholesterol mg/100ml) Before	After	% change
Whole milk	2 l	8	213	202*	–5
Skimmed milk	2 l	8	220	188**	–15
Butter	113 g	7	197	231*	+17
Calcium (as gluconate)	2.4 g	7	214	218	+2
Cottage cheese	800 g	6	221	229	+4
Lactose	100 g	10	200	190	–5
Cheese (Leicestershire)	220 g	7	210	214	+2
Whey (Leicestershire cheese)	2 l	6	196	201	+2
Cream	160 g	9	198	202	+2

* $P<0.05$, ** $P<0.01$

This new evidence may explain why the Masai of central Africa (Uganda, Tanzania and Kenya) who live almost exclusively on milk, drinking up to four litres/day have abnormally-low serum cholesterol (135 mg/100 ml) and a low incidence of coronary heart disease. The suggestion that the Masai drink fermented milk (yoghurt) rather than fresh (Mann, 1977*a*), and that the former contains a factor which decreases serum cholesterol, is non-proven. In experimental studies, yoghurt is no more active in lowering serum cholesterol than the milk from which it is made (Howard & Marks, 1979).

The 'milk factor' has so far not been identified. Milk contains large quantities of calcium, and although compounds containing this element have been reported to lower serum cholesterol, feeding the same quantity of calcium as in the milk had no effect. Likewise, the small effect produced by lactose was insufficient to account for the magnitude of the effect (Table 2).

The lack of effect of cheese whey and lactose indicates that the factor is not lactose. Rather surprisingly, cream and cheese also had no effect on serum cholesterol, in contrast to butterfat in which the expected rise occurred. This suggests that the hypocholesterolaemic factor may be present in the cell membranes surrounding the fat globules.

An alternative hypothesis is that when the quantities of dairy products consumed are large, the relative amounts of other components of the diet may be diminished. It can be argued that the cholesterol-lowering effect of milk may be due to a general reduction in saturated-fat intake and other dietary changes. This appears unlikely when the fat and calorie content of butter, cheese and cream are compared.

There is no evidence that any dairy product other than butter is hypercholesterolaemic. Malmros & Wigand (1957) carried out well-designed and executed experiments in Swedish volunteers. After consuming their normal diet for several weeks they were asked to consume 40 per cent of energy as milk fat (a mixture of milk, cheese, cream and butter). This diet gave a decrease in serum cholesterol from baseline values (although the authors claimed milk fat increased serum cholesterol in their discussion). It might be possible eventually to obtain the factor in a sufficiently concentrated and active form such that its addition to butter would counteract the hypercholesterolaemic effect of butter fat.

(iii) Mechanism of action of dietary fat

(a) Serum lipids

Despite attempts by several investigators to elucidate the mechanism by which dietary fat affects serum cholesterol, the problem is unsolved. Moore *et al.* (1968) claimed that polyunsaturated oils increased the faecal excretion of bile acids which provides a major route by which cholesterol is excreted (via metabolism in the liver). However, Grundy & Ahrens (1970), in isotopic balance studies, refuted this evidence and gave data to support the view that polyunsaturated fatty acids redistributed cholesterol from the serum to the tissue. It is likely that both mechanisms operate.

Even if one accepts this is the case, the reason why different fats change lipid metabolism is obscure. Until more is known on the subject, it may be impossible to emplain why butter raises serum cholesterol but whole milk does not.

(b) Thrombosis

An alternative explanation is that dietary fat can cause an increase in thrombosis, and it is this effect which is of importance in coronary heart disease. There is some experimental evidence in animals for this view. Butter and other saturated fats cause thrombosis in rats fed a very abnormal diet which rendered them extremely hypercholesterolaemic (Howard & Gresham, 1968). Likewise, Hornstra (1975) has demonstrated that the onset of occlusion in aortic cannulae in living rats is delayed by giving linoleic acid. This evidence is particularly convincing since polyunsaturated fats are precursors of prostaglandin E_1, a powerful inhibitor of platelet aggregation. In man, saturated fats can promote platelet aggregation and decrease fibrinolysis (Renaud, 1977; Nordoy & Rodset, 1971). Because *in-vitro* tests to investigate thrombotic tendency cannot be directly extrapolated to the *in-vivo* situation, many of the results obtained are of limited value. Despite this criticism, there is a strong possibility that saturated fat can influence thrombosis.

(iv) Experimental evidence for dietary fat hypothesis

If the dietary fat hypothesis is true, then the logical step should be to advise populations who live on a high saturated-fat diet to modify their diet accordingly. So far, the evidence that a change in diet can affect cardiovascular disease is not entirely convincing.

Two trials which have examined the effect of a so called 'prudent diet' (high polyunsaturated, low saturated fat and low cholesterol) on the morbidity and mortality of patients with coronary heart disease have given equivocal results. In a trial in Oslo, Leren (1966) found that in 412 subjects lowering serum cholesterol by 14 per cent did not affect the incidence of sudden deaths. However, the number of coronary events without death were significantly reduced (Table 3). Likewise in a trial with 373 patients, in which soya-bean oil was employed (Morris *et al.*, 1968), the difference in serum cholesterol between experimental subjects and controls was 16 per cent and no difference in death rate was established.

There have been several trials in which a 'prudent' diet has been examined as a prospective study in healthy populations (Christakis *et al.*, 1966; Turpeinen *et. al.*, 1968; Dayton *et al.*, 1969). Whilst the incidence of coronary events has been statistically reduced, the overall affect on mortality was not striking. Table 3 shows the results of three trials in New York, Helsinki and Los Angeles. First the mean difference in serum cholesterol achieved by diet was not large, being 25-50 mg/100 ml (10-15 per cent). A clearcut and statistical reduction in deaths from coronary heart disease was achieved only in the Los Angeles trial but overall mortality was not affected, there being more deaths from cancer in the experimental group.

There is some evidence that lowering serum cholesterol by drugs can be effective. For instance, in a recent study 10 000 people were treated for seven years with the drug clofibrate which lowered serum cholesterol by 9 per cent (Oliver *et al.*, 1978). The incidence of symptoms but not mortality from coronary heart disease, was decreased by 20 per cent. However, more deaths occurred from other causes in the clofibrate-treated group so the results are difficult to interpret.

Another trial with the anion exchange resin colestipol gave a more positive result (Dorr, Martin & Freyburger, 1974). This drug acts by combining with bile acids in the gastro-intestinal tract. Over 500 patients with pre-existing coronary heart disease were treated with either placebo or drug. The number of deaths was greatly reduced in the drug-treated group, and the serum cholesterol was decreased by 15 per cent.

(v) Controversial aspects

Whilst most would agree that there is a direct correlation between coronary heart disease and serum cholesterol, the widescale manipulation of the public's diet to achieve a reduction is highly controversial, and has been the subject of discussion of several committees. The (US) Council on Foods and Nutrition

Table 3. Effect on diet on mortality from coronary heart disease

Type of prevention trial	Place	Total no. of subjects		Serum cholesterol (m/100ml)		No. of deaths from coronary heart disease		No. of subjects with relapses	
		Experimental	Control	Experimental	Control	Experimental	Control	Experimental	Control
Primary	New York[1]	941	457	225	250	Not available*	Not available	17	32
	Helsinki[2]	313	241	217	268	7	10	17	30
	Los Angeles[3]	424	422	186	232	18	27	54	71
Secondary	London[4]	194	199	221	258	27	25	47	60
	Oslo[5]	206	206	239	283	27	27	64	90

[1] Christakis *et al.* (1966), [2] Turpeinen *et al.* (1968), [3] Dayton *et al.* (1969), [4] Morris *et al.* (1968), [5] Leren (1966)

* No significance in total deaths.

(1972), after considering the evidence, recommended that: (1) Measurement of the plasma-lipid profile, particularly of plasma cholesterol, should become a routine part of health maintenance; (2) Persons falling into a risk category (above 220 mg/100 ml serum cholesterol) should be given dietary advice. In practice, this entails substituting polyunsaturated vegetable oils for part of the saturated fat in the diet; (3) High priority should be given to the conduct of studies that will determine reliably the extent to which modification of plasma lipids by diet can reduce the risk of developing coronary heart disease.

In the United Kingdom, two committees meeting within two years of each other and examining the same evidence, gave slightly different views. A joint working party of the Royal College of Physicians of London and the British Cardiac Society (1976) approved of a reduction in saturated fat (from 40 to 35 per cent total calories) and agreed with the Americans that foods high in polyunsaturated fats should offer a partial replacement. The Department of Health and Social Security Advisory Panel (DHSS, 1974) recommended that the amount of saturated fat in the diet should be reduced, but a recommendation could not be made to increase the intake of polyunsaturated acid 'since the evidence of such a change being beneficial was lacking.'

However, not everyone shares the above opinions. Whilst agreeing with the premise that a high serum cholesterol is a risk factor, Reiser (1978) was unconvinced that a serum cholesterol below 250 mg/100 ml is of any importance. He based his argument chiefly on the results of the US National Cooperative Pooling project which showed that there is no difference in death rate from coronary heart disease in the range 175-250 mg/100 ml, whereas above this figure death rate is markedly increased. Reiser (1978) felt that advice to the population in general, as opposed to those who have been found to have high serum cholesterol levels, is of little value. However, this ignores the fact that different populations with low risk (eg the Japanese and the Masai) have very low serum-cholesterol levels and that a value below 175 mg/100 ml might be even more beneficial. Also the Framingham study showed a linear risk down to a cholesterol level of 180 mg/100 ml. In a review of data from mainland China (Cheng, 1973), the mean normal serum cholesterol was reported to be 136 mg/100 ml and 190 mg/100 ml in coronary-heart-disease patients.

George Mann (1977*b*) has a number of objections to the dietary fat hypothesis. First, in the Framingham and many other studies, no correlation was found between the saturated-fat intake as measured by the 24-hour recall method and serum cholesterol. This criticism can be countered by pointing out the inaccuracy of this particular method of dietary assessment over the long term. Secondly, Mann (1977*b*) claims that the mortality trends over the last 30 years do not give any support for the theory. However, this is not apparently substantiated by the facts. For between 1970-1975 there has been a reduction of 35 per cent in butter consumption and the intake of polyunsaturated fatty acids has risen from 7 to 15 per cent in the USA, as a result of public education (National Center for Health Statistics, 1978), and this has been associated with a 20 per cent decrease in the incidence of coronary heart disease and a decline in serum cholesterol. Whilst this evidence is consistent with the dietary fat hypothesis, change in cigarette-smoking habits and an increase in physical exercise may also be implicated.

With such a highly controversial subject it is difficult to be dogmatic. Whilst there is some positive evidence to implicate saturated fat, and a reduction in its intake would not cause any ill effects, the convincing demonstration that a change in diet would be beneficial is still awaited. Such a trial would involve large numbers of subjects, be very expensive, and would take many years to complete. The main problem is whether and how the public should be advised to change their dietary habits. Certainly those with an abnormally high serum cholesterol (>250 mg/100 ml) are at a greater risk than others, and any dietary advice may be of greater value in these cases.

3. Sucrose

The widely publicised hypothesis that sucrose is a major factor in coronary heart disease has been examined by many authors (eg see Chapter 6) and found to be unacceptable; the chief arguments against it were summarised by Ancel Keys (1971). The epidemiological evidence is rather weak. There are several countries with a very high intake of sucrose with low incidence of coronary heart disease. There has not been a large increase in sugar consumption since the beginning of the century. Despite claims to the contrary, men who have had coronary heart disease do not consume more sugar than others. Sucrose can cause a transient rise in serum triglycerides, but there is a general lack of supporting experimental evidence in man or animals to explain how sucrose could be implicated. For those ardent devotees of the hypothesis, however, an effect on platelet aggregation and thrombosis offers a feasible mechanism (Yudkin, Szanto & Kakkar, 1969).

4. Alcohol

The effects of alcohol vary with the quantity taken and its duration. Also some individuals are more sensitive to change than others. Moderate drinking causes an increase in VLDL (Taskinen & Nikkila, 1977), and serum triglycerides, but not cholesterol or LDL, are elevated (Sirtori *et al.*, 1972). HDL-cholesterol is raised, the magnitude of the effect increasing with the quantity drunk, up to a 20 per cent mean increase being observed. If a raised HDL-cholesterol is protective than alcohol could have beneficial side-effects (Castelli, 1977).

5. Protein

Since the beginning of the century there has been no change in total consumption or quality of protein consumed in Great Britain (DHSS, 1974). Thus, it seems unlikely that protein plays a major involvement in coronary heart disease in this country. If one compares different countries there is a correlation between incidence and animal protein consumption, but it is weaker than for animal fat (Connor & Connor, 1972).

The strongest evidence is found in the rabbit. This species fed a diet containing semi-purified ingredients develops a high serum cholesterol in two weeks and atherosclerosis in three months. The main active constituent is animal protein (eg casein). Substitution of vegetable (eg soya) for animal protein prevents the disease (Carroll & Hamilton, 1975). Likewise in man, significant reductions in serum cholesterol have been reported in hypercholesterolaemic patients given a soya-bean protein 'isolate' (Sirtori *et al.*, 1977). Whilst the change of protein could be the explanation, the soya product contained, in addition, 15-20 per cent other substances which might equally have produced the observed effect. This criticism can also be applied to another experiment in which an intake of 100 g/day animal protein was changed to 25 per cent/day vegetable protein from cereals and legumes (Olsen *et al.*, 1958). A reduction in serum cholesterol was observed, but this could easily be due to the increased fibre intake.

6. Fibre

This topic has been covered briefly in chapter 5. In summary, hydrophilic indigestible polysaccharides such as pectin and guar gum have a modest effect on serum cholesterol (about 30 g/day produces a 15 per cent lowering). Such effects are not seen with wheat fibre, and that from oatmeal has only a small effect. The hydrophilic fibres are particularly prone to attack by the intestinal bacteria, and it could be that the variation in response is due to individual differences in the destruction of the fibre by bacteria (Southgate, 1978).

Legumes such as peas and beans lower serum cholesterol but it is not known if this activity is related to the high content of indigestible polysaccharides (Grande, Anderson & Keys, 1965).

Epidemiological evidence for the involvement of fibre is fairly strong. There is a strong negative correlation between incidence of coronary heart disease and fibre intake in different countries (Trowell, 1977). In a study lasting a period of 20 years, Morris and colleagues carefully measured the food intake of a group of over 300 men (Morris *et al.*, 1977). As shown in Table 4 (Morris, Marr & Clayton, 1978), the deaths from coronary heart disease were considerably less

Table 4. Daily dietary-fibre intake and incidence of coronary heart disease (Morris, J.N., Marr, J.W. & Clayton, D.G., 1978)

Dietary fibre: thirds of distribution of men*	*(a)* **Total dietary fibre**		*(b)* **Fibre from fruit, vegetables, pulses, and nuts**		*(c)* **Fibre from cereals**	
	g/man/day	Cases of CHD	g/man/day	Cases of CHD	g/man/day	Cases of CHD
Low third	5.6 - 15.4	22	0.6 - 6.9	14	2.0 - 7.1	25
Middle third	13.8 - 19.0	16	6.1 - 9.0	18	6.4 - 9.7	15
High third	16.9 - 56.1	7	8.3 - 26.5	13	8.4 - 34.2	5

* Thirds composed of 112, 113 and 112 men respectively, classified according to thirds of dietary fibre intake in each occupation (see Morris *et al.*, 1977)

Men were aged 30-67 at initial survey. Cases of CHD up to 70 years.

in those with a high-fibre intake. This applied only to fibre from cereals (chiefly from wheat) and not fruit and vegetables. The changes were not associated with differences in serum cholesterol. This result would indicate that cereal fibre has a protective effect, and its mechanism of action might be concerned with a factor other than serum lipids, for instance, prevention of thrombosis.

7. Vitamins

Several claims have been made over the years that specific vitamins, either in deficiency or excess, are of importance (Truswell, 1978). In almost all cases further investigations proved negative, for instance, in the case of biotin, vitamin C (see Chapter 3) and vitamin E.

The case for vitamin D is fairly strong (Linden, 1974). Over-dosage can promote calcification of the media of the arterial wall of the coronary arteries, which then predisposes the intima to lipid deposition. Large doses also produce a small increase in serum cholesterol.

There is cause for concern over the excessive fortification of foods by vitamin D.

8. Minerals and the water factor

Attention was first drawn to a possible relationship between vascular disease and water supply in Japan where there appeared to be a direct relationship between deaths from cerebral haemorrhage and the sulphate-bicarbonate ratio of the river water (Kobayashi, 1957). This report led Schroeder (1960) to study death rates in the United States in relation to the drinking water. Rather surprisingly, he found that in 163 of the larger cities, the death rate from coronary heart disease was highest in those areas with *soft* water. He therefore concluded that some factor was present in drinking water associated with its softness which accentuated mortality from two major cardiovascular diseases – cerebral haemorrhage in Japan and coronary heart disease in the USA. Schroeder's statistical findings have been confirmed elsewhere, notably in the United Kingdom, Holland, Sweden and Canada.

In the United Kingdom, Crawford, Gardner & Morris (1968) showed that in 61 county boroughs of England and Wales with a population of over 80 000 in 1961, the harder the local drinking water and the more calcium it contained, the lower was the death rate in middle and early old age; this was particularly so for cardiovascular mortality. Chemical studies of trace elements in water from consumer's taps showed none at a concentration which could be considered toxic either in towns with very soft or very hard water.

The death rates in Glasgow for cardiovascular disease is about the highest in Britain (654 per 100 000 for people aged 45-64 years) and the city has a very soft water supply. Greater London has a very hard drinking water and similar deaths (440 per 100 000) are approximately two-thirds those in Glasgow.

Probably the most interesting report is from Lincolnshire (Robertson, 1968), where a rise in death rate from cardiovascular disease over seven years occurred in Scunthorpe, when the water supply was artificially softened (Fig. 5). Nearby Grimsby has exactly the same water supply but unsoftened. Scunthorpe has 27 per cent more deaths than Grimsby. Moreover, while death rates are still rising in Scunthorpe they are falling slightly in Grimsby. The local water board have taken the unusual step of doubling the calcium content of the town's water supply and have given up using the water softener.

There is no clear evidence as yet as to what is present or missing in soft water that makes it so deleterious. Analysis of the water supplied in England and Wales showed that hard water contained greater quantities of calcium, magnesium and

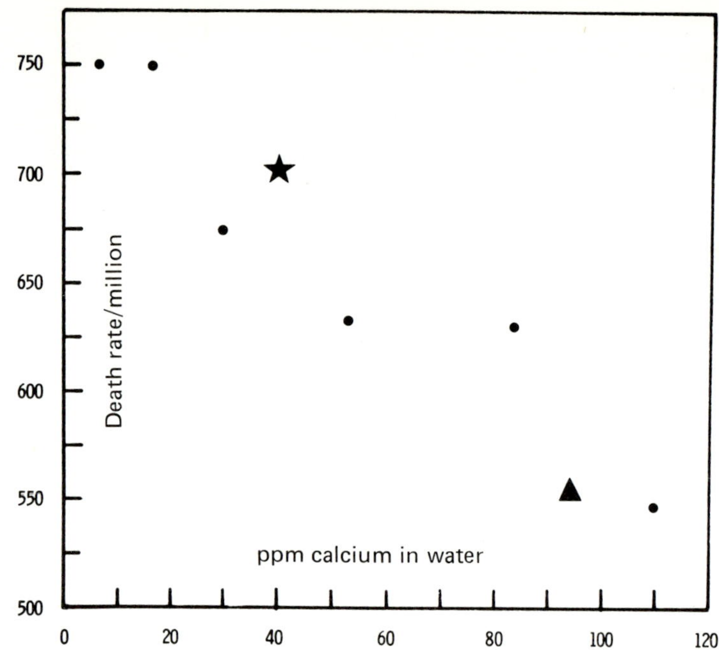

Fig. 5. Deaths from cardiovascular disease in the United Kingdom Data from Crawford *et al.* (1968) and Robertson (1968).Symbols: ● = from Crawford, ★= Scunthorpe (softened and ▲ = Grimsby (hard)

sodium, but that some other metals such as iron, zinc, lead, tin, nickel and chromium were the same as for soft water (Schroeder, LeRiche & MacKay, 1969). However, analysis of water at reservoirs can be very misleading. Soft water is notoriously acidic and corrosive to metal pipes, and it could be that some toxic contaminant is introduced. Support for this idea is the finding that in England the lead content of rib bones was considerably higher in soft-water than in hard-water areas. Although lead has not been specifically linked with cardiovascular deaths, cadmium, a contaminant of zinc used in galvanizing, does cause hypertension in rats, and Schroeder *et al.* (1960) have suggested this might be the possible link between deaths from cerebral haemorrhage in Japan and coronary heart disease elsewhere in the Western world. This hypothesis is attractive, since it explains a number of other confusing factors. For instance, in Toronto (Anderson, 1969), the higher death rate in soft water areas was found to be due to sudden death, possibly associated with hypertension. Also, in a study in Glasgow, Crawford & Crawford (1967) found no greater incidence of stenosis and diseases of the coronary arteries than in parts of England where the water is hard.

Other minerals which have been suggested as important are calcium, chromium and silicon. Calcium causes an increase in the excretion of bile acids by forming insoluble bile-acid salts. This leads to a lowering of plasma cholesterol and in some studies 1.5/g calcium/day caused a significant depression (Yacowitz, Fleischman & Beirenbaum, 1965). However, it is doubtful if the calcium content of hard water is sufficient to cause any demonstrable effect.

Chromium and silicon are other metals which have been shown to be hypocholesterolaemic in rats (Truswell, 1978), but their effects in man seems uncertain.

In view of the importance of the problem there seems little direct evidence to pinpoint any of the suggested factors. So far, experimental work in animals has been disappointing. In pigs (Howard, Jennings & Gresham, 1967), no difference was found in the extent of atherosclerosis in animals given water of different hardness. However, the commercial diets used were heavily fortified with minerals and could have obscured any effect.

Conclusions

There is much evidence to implicate several nutritional factors in the aetiology of coronary heart disease, but the picture is not clear. Given that elevated serum lipids are risk factors, the extent to which the different nutrients such as dietary fat, carbohydrates, fibre, affect individuals and the way that the different nutrients interact is uncertain. Clear-cut prospective studies to determine the effect of nutrients on the incidence of coronary heart disease are badly needed.

Likewise, the ability of nutrients to damage the arterial wall and promote thrombosis is not fully explained. The main problem here is the difficulty in devising suitable experimental models and then extrapolating the results to man.

References

Anderson, T.W. (1969): *New Engl. J. Med.* **280**, 805.

Anitschkow, N. (1933): In *Arteriosclerosis,* ed E.V. Cowdry, p. 271. New York: MacMillan.

Assman, G. & Schaefer, H-E. (1978): In *Int. Conf. on Atherosclerosis,* ed L.A. Carlson, R. Paoletti, C.R. Sirtori & G. Webber, pp. 97-101. New York: Raven.

Baird, I.M. & Howard, A.N. Editors (1969): *Obesity: Medical and scientific aspects.* Edinburgh: Livingstone.

Bray, G.A. Editor (1978): *Recent advances in obesity research:* 2, London: Newman.

Bronte-Stewart, B. (1958): *Br. Med. Bull.* **14**, 243.

Bronte-Stewart, B., Keys, A. & Brock, J.F. (1955): *Lancet* **2**, 100.

Carlson, L.A. & Bottinger, L.E. (1972): *Lancet* **1**, 865.

Carroll, K.K. & Hamilton, R.M.G. (1975): *J. Fd Sci.* **40**, 18.

Castelli, W.P. (1977): *Lancet* **2**, 153.

Cheng, T.O. (1973): *Ann. Int. Med.* **78**, 285.

Christakis, G. *et al.* (1966): *Am. J. Publ. Hlth* **56**, 299.

Connor, W.E., Hodges, R.E. & Bleiler, R.E. (1961): *J. Clin. Invest.* **40**, 894.

Connor, W.E. & Connor, S.L. (1972): *Prev. Med.* **1**, 49.

Council on Foods and Nutrition (1972): *J. Am. Med. Ass.* **222**, 1647.

Crawford, T. & Crawford, M.D. (1967): *Lancet* **1**, 229.

Crawford, M.D., Gardner, M.J. & Morris, J.N. (1968): *Lancet* **1**, 747.

Dam, H. *et al.* (1970): *Z. Ernahrungswissenschaft* **10**, 178.

Dayton, S. (1972): In *Pharmacological control of lipid metabolism,* ed W.L. Holmes, R. Paoletti & D. Kritchevsky, p. 245. New York: Plenum.

Dayton, S. *et al.* (1969): *Am. Heart Ass. Monogr. No. 25.*

Department of Health and Social Security (1974): *Diet and coronary heart disease.* Rep. Hlth Soc. Subj. No. 7. London: HMSO.

Dorr, E.A., Martin, W.B. & Freyburger, W.A. (1974): In *Proceedings 5th Int. Symp. on drugs affecting lipid metabolism,* Milan.

Grande, F., Anderson, J.T. & Keys, A. (1965): *J. Nutr.* **86**, 213.

Grundy, S.M. & Ahrens, E.H. (1970): *J. Clin. Invest.* **49**, 1135.

Hornstra, G. (1975): In *Role of fats in human nutrition,* ed A.J. Vergroesen. London: Academic Press.
Howard, A.N. editor (1975): *Recent advances in obesity research: 1.* London: Newman.
Howard, A.N. (1977): *Atherosclerosis* 27, 383.
Howard, A.N. & Gresham, G.A. (1968): *Int. Z. Vitaminforschung* **38**, 545.
Howard, A.N., Jennings, I.W. & Gresham, G.A. (1967): *Path. Microbiol.* **30**, 676.
Howard, A.N. & Marks, J. (1977): *Lancet* 2, 275.
Howard, A.N. & Marks, J. (1979): *Lancet* 2, 957.
Kannel, W.B., Castelli, W.P., Gordron, T. & McNamara, P.M. (1971): *Ann. Intern. Med.* 74, 1.
Keys, A. (1967): *J. Am. Diet. Ass.* **51**, 508.
Keys, A. (1970): *Circulation* **41**, Suppl. 1, 1.
Keys, A. (1971): *Atherosclerosis* **14**, 193.
Keys, A., Anderson, J.T. & Grande, F. (1965): *Metabolism* **14**, 776.
Keys, A., Mickelson, O., Miller, E.D. & Chapman, C.B. (1950): *Science* **112**, 79.
Kobayashi, J. (1957): *Ber. d.Ohara. Inst. Landwirsch Biol.* **11**, 12.
Kritchevsky, D. (1958): *Cholesterol* New York: Wiley.
Leren, P. (1966): *Acta Med. Scand.* Suppl. 466.
Lewis, B. (1978): *J. Roy. Soc. Med.* **71**, 809-818.
Linden, V. (1974): *Br. Med. J.* **3**, 647.
Malmros, H. (1950): *Acta Med. Scand. Suppl.* **246**, 316.
Malmros, H. & Wigand, G. (1957): *Lancet* 2, 1.
Mann, G.V. (1977*a*): *Atherosclerosis* **26**, 335.
Mann, G.V. (1977*b*): *New Engl. J. Med.* **297**, 644.
Messinger, W.J., Poroswiska, Y. & Steele, J.M. (1950): *Archs Int. Med.* **86**, 189.
Miller, G.J. & Miller, N.E. (1975): *Lancet* **1**, 16.
Miller, N.E., Forde, O.H., Thelle, D.S. & Mjos, O.D. (1977): *Lancet* 2, 977.
Mistry, P., Nicoll, A., Niehaus, C., Christie, I., James, E. & Lewis, B. (1976): *Circulation* **54**, Suppl. 2, 178.
Moore, R.B., Anderson, J.T., Taylor, H.L., Keys, A. & Frantz, I. (1968): *J. Clin. Invest.* **47**, 1517.
Morris, J.N. *et al.* (1968): *Lancet* 2, 693.
Morris, J.N., Marr, J.W. & Clayton, D.G. (1977): *Br. Med. J.* 2, 1307.
Morris, J.N., Marr, J.W. & Clayton, D.G. (1978): *J. Plant Fds* 3, 45-54.
National Center for Health Statistics (1978): *Vital and health statistics.* Hyattsville, Md: Publ. Hlth Serv. DHEW.
Nødry, A. & Rødset, J.M. (1971): *Acta Med. Scand.* **190**, 27.
Office of population censuses and surveys (1978): *Mortality statistics 1976, Cause,* DH2, No. 3. London: HMSO.
Oliver, M.F. *et al.* (1978): *Br. Heart J.* **40**, 1069.
Olsen, R.E. *et al.* (1958): *Am. J. Clin. Nutr.* **6**, 310.
Pelkonen, R., Nikkila, E.A., Koskinen, S., Perittinen, K. & Sarna, S. (1977): *Br. Med. J.* 2, 1185.
Porter, M.W., Yamanaka, W., Carlson, S.D. & Flynn, M.A. (1977): *Am. J. Clin. Nutr.* **30**, 490.
Reiser, R. (1978): *Am. J. Clin. Nutr.* **31**, 865.
Renaud, S. (1977): *Biblio. Nutr. Diet.* **25**, 92.
Royal College of Physicians of London and British Cardiac Society jt working party (1976): *J. Roy. Coll. Physns.* **10**, 213.
Roberston, J.S. (1968): *Lancet* 2, 348.
Schettler, G. (1950): *Klin. Wschr.* **28**, 565.
Schroeder, H.A. (1960): *J. Am. Med. Ass.* **172**, 1902.
Schroeder, H.W., Le Riche, H.W. & McKay, J.S. (1969): *New. Engl. J. Med.* **280**, 836.
Sirtori, C.R. *et al.* (1972): *Lancet* 2, 820.
Sirtori, C.R. *et al.* (1977): *Lancet* **1**, 275.
Southgate, D.A.T. (1978): *J. Plant Fds* 3, 9-19.
Taskinen, M.R. & Nikkila, E.A. (1977): *Acta Med. Scand.* **202**, 173.
Trowell, H. (1977): *Am. J. Clin. Nutr.* **25**, 926.
Truswell, A.S. (1978): *Am. J. Clin. Nutr.* **31**, 977.
Turpeinen, O. *et al.* (1968): *Am. J. Clin. Nutr.* **21**, 255.
Worth, R.M. *et al.* (1975): *Am. J. Epidemiol.* **102**, 481.
Yacowitz, H., Fleischman, A.A. & Beirenabum, A.A. (1965):
Yudkin, J., Szanto, S. & Kakkar, V.V. (1969): *Postgrad. Med. J.* **45**, 608.

9

Nutritional deficiencies in the elderly

A.N. Exton-Smith.

Introduction

Although frank malnutrition has been largely eliminated from most sections of the population of the United Kindom it is still occasionally found amongst the elderly. The First Report of the Panel on the Nutrition of the Elderly (Department of Health and Social Security, 1970) stated that 'there is little doubt that more is known of the nutritional state of our nation than of any other in the world, but in relation to the elderly the evidence is still inadequate'. The Panel recommended that field surveys on which the Department of Health and its collaborators have already embarked should be complemented by longitudinal studies designed to detect changes in nutritional intakes with age and to determine the relationship between nurition and health in old age.

Nutritional surveys

Most of the nutritional surveys which have been made of the elderly population have been on the basis of cross-sectional or point-of-time studies. Thus differences between the old and young can be established when measurements made on groups of individuals of various ages are compared. These surveys have usually revealed that a proportion of subjects have very low intakes of certain nutrients. To assess the effects on health on these low intakes, serial investigations on the same individual are required. Moreover these longitudinal studies, as they are called, are the only means of clearly identifying the changes which are due to ageing. Ideally the repeated measurements should be made on the same person at standardised intervals over as long a period as possible; for obvious reasons there have been very few studies of this kind.

Cross-sectional studies

There have been a number of nutritional surveys of random samples of the elderly population at home and of old people in hospitals and residential homes. In a survey sponsored by the King Edward's Hospital Fund (Exton-Smith & Stanton, 1965) an investigation was made of the diets of old people living alone at home in two north London boroughs. The group selected was 60 women whose ages ranged from 70-80 years (with the exception of three aged 89, 90 and 94 years). The mean daily intakes of nutrients were satisfactory and are shown in Table 1 below.

Table 1. Mean daily intakes of nutrients of women in the eigth decade

Total energy	1890 kcal	Calcium	860mg
	7.9 MJ	Iron	9.9mg
Protein	57g	Vitamin C	37mg
Fat	74g	Vitamin D	135iu
Carbohydrate	221g		

Only a few instances of nutritional deficiency were revealed by the survey. There was, however, a striking correlation between diet and health; nearly all the subjects whose diet was better than average were judged on clinical assessment to be better than average in health. This does not necessarily mean that good diet is responsible for good health, since the reverse might equally be true in that better health and physical activity might be associated with good appetite and a larger intake of food.

When 60 subjects were arranged in groups according to their ages there was found to be a striking decrease in intakes of all nutrients with advancing age. The percentage falls in intake for subjects in their late 70s compared with those in their early 70s are shown in Table 2 below.

Table 2. Cross-sectional study: fall in intake of total energy and nutrients during the eigth decade (%)

Total energy	19
Protein	24
Fat	30
Carbohydrate	8
Calcium	18
Iron	29
Vitamin C	31

In spite of the considerable reduction in nutrient intake with age there seemed to be little alteration in the quality of the diet. Thus the percentage of energy derived from protein was 12.2 per cent for the subjects in their early 70s and 11.4 per cent for those in their late 70s.

This point-of-time study reveals age differences which might be the result of several factors:

(1) True age changes affecting all individuals and leading to a reduction in physiological requirements. It is known that lean body mass and basal metabolic rate decrease with age (Allen, Anderson & Langham, 1960).

(2) Reduction in appetite or energy expenditure in some of the subjects due to the development of disease or physical disabilities as they enter the second half of the eighth decade. Sheldon (1948) has drawn attention to the striking increase in prevalence of incapacity in the elderly population after the age of 75.

(3) Secular differences between the two groups in that lifelong dietary pattern of the old group may have been different from that of the early 70s group. Indeed

it is possible that the dietary pattern may have been a factor responsible for the longevity of those who reach extreme old age.

(4) The failure of certain individuals, notably the obese, to reach extreme old age. The late 70s group, being thinner, would be expected to have a lower dietary intake.

From this study it was impossible to ascertain the relative importance of these factors and it was therefore decided to conduct a follow-up study of the 60 elderly women to form a longitudinal investigation.

Longitudinal studies

Twenty-two of the 60 women who participated in the first King Edward's Hospital Fund Survey were followed-up six-and-a-half years later (Stanton & Exton-Smith, 1970). It was found that for those subjects who maintained their health (as assessed on clinical examination and by a scoring system recording physical disabilities) the intakes of nutrients in the two surveys were remarkably similar. But, for those women whose health had declined, there was a considerable fall in intake, amounting to 20 per cent for protein and 17 per cent for energy.

From this limited study it was concluded that nutrient intakes in old age are usually maintained provided the person remains active and fit. It was also evident that physical disabilities are often responsible for declining intakes in old age. It is necessary in this age group, at least when assessing nutrient requirements, to include medical examinations of the subjects when carrying out dietary surveys (Exton-Smith, 1970).

One of the first longitudinal studies to assess the nutritional status of the aged was carried out in San Mateo, California. The initial survey on 577 healthy subjects lived in their own homes (Gillum & Morgan, 1955). When the data from this first survey were analysed on a cross-sectional basis by comparing the intakes of the subjects in three age groups, namely 55-64, 65-74, 75 years and over, it was found that there was a progressive fall in intakes with age, especially after 75, similar to that found in the first survey of the King Edward's Hospital Fund. Further studies were conducted, four, six and 14 years after the original survey and there were 141 participants in all four surveys (Chope & Breslow, 1956; Steinkamp, Cohen & Walsh, 1965). Although a reduction in food intake after the age of 75 occurred there was no significant difference between the four studies in the proportion of energy contributed by carbohydrate, protein and fat, for any of the groups. Moreover, there was little alteration with age in individual intakes of animal protein, thus those subjects with low intakes in 1948 tended to maintain the same pattern through to 1962. When interpreting these studies, we are still not able to determine whether the lifelong nutrition pattern of those who reach extreme old age has contributed to their longevity, or whether their heredity which has enabled them to survive has also in some manner characterised their nutrition (Watkin, 1968).

The occurrence of malnutrition

Malnutrition has been defined as a disturbance of form or function due to lack of (or excess of) energy or of one or more nutrients (Department of Health and

Social Security, 1970). This definition includes both under-nutrition and obesity. In elderly women obesity can present a problem, for example, by giving rise to difficulties in rehabilitation of the patient who has suffered the effects of a cerebrovascular accident. In a survey of a random sample of the elderly population of Wolverhampton (Sheldon, 1948) one-quarter of the women over the age of 85 were obese; thus for women obesity does not necessarily prevent the attainment of extreme old age. For men, however, obesity has a poor prognosis and few men who are more than 20 per cent overweight live beyond the age of 75 (Anderson, 1967). Moreover, obesity usually results from lifelong faulty eating habits and in this respect differs from undernutrition which often arises from environmental and physical factors operating for the first time in later life.

Primary and secondary causes of malnutrition
In this review consideration will be given to common types of nutritional deficiency which affect old people; the factors responsible are summarised in Table 3 below.

Table 3. Primary and secondary causes of malnutrition in old age

Primary	**Secondary**
Ignorance	Impaired appetite
Social isolation	Masticatory inefficiency
Physical disability	Malabsorption
Mental disturbance	Alcoholism
Iatrogenic	Drugs
Poverty	Increased requirements

There is not always a very clear distinction between primary and secondary causes and very often several factors operate together to produce malnutrition in one individual.

Ignorance. The King Edward's Hospital Fund Survey (Exton-Smith & Stanton, 1965) showed that ignorance of the simple facts of nutrition is prevalent amongst elderly women. Many of them had learnt what little they knew about food purchasing and cooking from their mothers in childhood; articles in popular magazines and talks on the radio had little influence. It is likely that, in men, ignorance is even more prevalent, especially in certain sections of the elderly male population. Thus a man who is recently widowed may have to fend for himself for the first time and he may have little idea of what constitutes a balanced diet. Widower's scurvy is seen in the man living mostly on packaged foods, tea, bread, butter and jam.

Social isolation. For many old people living alone in social isolation with few human contacts there is loss of interest sometimes amounting to apathy and consequent neglect in the preparation of food. What food is eaten is usually taken in the form of snacks. The Stockport Survey (Brockington & Lempert, 1967) of the social needs of the over 80s showed that dietary intake was related to the number of outside interests of old people. Dietary intake was found to be better in those old people who eat at clubs in the company of others.

Physical disabilities. Elderly persons with locomotive disorders such as hemiplegia and arthritis may have difficulty in getting and preparing food. This applies particularly to the housebound people living alone without adequate support.

Mental disturbances. The unmet medical and social needs of the elderly are believed to be greatest in those with psychiatric disorders (Stokoe, 1965). Malnutrition is also common in this group which consists mainly of people suffering from organic brain syndromes and confusional states. Moreover, Fowlie, Cohen & Anand (1963) have shown a clear association between malnutrition and depressive illness, which leads to a disinclination to obtain, prepare, and even in severe cases, to eat food.

Iatrogenic. Sometimes a badly planned dietary regime leads to malnutrition, expecially when it is continued by the patient for much longer than necessary. Thus a number of cases of scurvy have been reported in patients having a 'gastric' diet for peptic ulcer, since this is often deficient in vitamin C. Investigations have shown that the vitamin C status of peptic ulcer patients, as measured by the leucocyte ascorbic acid levels, is frequently inferior to that of people without peptic ulceration.

Poverty. Many old people have to make a choice between spending money on food or fuel, and poverty is a factor to be considered in old age more often than in other age groups. The food eaten by pensioners is often dull, monotonous and tasteless. Brockington & Lempert (1967) showed that old people who are able to supplement their incomes from savings or income from a part-time occupation have a better diet than those whose sole financial means is the old-age pension.

Impaired appetite. Transitory impairment of appetite is common in old age. Thus even a respiratory infection can curtail food intake over a number of days and in a person whose nutrition is already marginal frank malnutrition may be precipitated.

Masticatory inefficiency. Although it is surprsing how many old people manage without teeth, a poor state of dentition or ill-fitting dentures often makes an individual select mushy foods consisting mainly of carbohydrate and the more nutritious foods requiring mastication are avoided. The intake of animal protein is particularly likely to be affected.

Malabsorption. Mild degrees of malabsorption are not uncommon in old people. In some cases this is due to bowel ischaemia, but the possibility of gluten sensitivity even after the age of 70 must be borne in mind. The absorption of fat and fat-soluble vitamins is mainly affected.

Alcohol and drugs. When the intake of alcohol is excessive, energy needs may be derived chiefly from this source and intake of certain nutrients greatly curtailed. The association between folic acid deficiency and the long-continued use of barbiturates and anti-convulsant drugs is well known. Secondary deficiency of the B group of vitamins may occur as the result of inadequate absorption in patients receiving anti-microbial drugs which alter the colonic flora.

Increased requirements. Negative nitrogen balance and the breakdown of tissue protein can occur in patients who are immobilised in bed for long periods, in those who suffer from long-continued pyrexia, and as a result of deep bed-sores with the loss of protein-rich fluid. The impairment of appetite which often accompanies these conditions is an additional factor.

Vulnerable groups

Several factors, both primary and secondary, often operate together to produce malnutrition in the individual. Sometimes these factors are inter-related; thus limited mobility, loneliness, social isolation and depression are all found in housebound old people and make them especially prone to malnutrition when they are receiving insufficient support from relatives, friends or the community.

In the survey of a random sample of the elderly population of Wolverhampton, Sheldon (1948) investigated the capacity for movement of old people. He found that 2.5 per cent were bedfast and a further 8.5 per cent had limitation of movement which restricted them to the house. He demonstrated a striking increase in disability with age; for the age group 60-64 years 1.5 per cent were housebound, but for those aged 85 and over no less than 32 per cent were confined to the house. Sheldon showed a clear relationship between loneliness and capacity for movement. The bedfast were the least lonely since they had constant human contacts derived from the need for nursing attention which of necessity had to be supplied to maintain them in their homes. On the other hand, the highest incidence of loneliness was found in those whose activities confined them to the house and it exceeded that found in the sample as a whole. Sheldon attributed this to the fact that many of these subjects were well enough to be left alone all day but were not capable of sufficient physical activity to keep them fully occupied.

Since 10 per cent of the elderly population are housebound (and this figure has been confirmed by the results of the nutrition surveys organised by the Department of Health and Social Security) there could be about three-quarters of a million housebound old people in Great Britain. Thus this section of the population represents the largest single group vulnerable to malnutrition. When the dietary and state of health of housebound old people were investigated by Exton-Smith, Stanton & Windsor (1972) the housebound were found to have nutrient intakes which are substantially lower than those of active old people of comparable age. Thus physical and mental disability in old age not only affect the mode of living of those afflicted but also lead to alterations in their dietary pattern and nutritional status.

Subclinical malnutrition

Special tests, including biochemical, haematological, and radiological investigations, often reveal small departures from normality and these can be related to the low intakes of certain nutrients. In younger persons the margin of safety is wide, but in old age homeostatic mechanisms are often impaired and the precarious physiological balance may be upset by the operation of medical and environmental hazards to which the elderly are prone. Frank malnutrition may be precipitated by such stress in those individuals whose nutrition is only marginally adequate (Exton- Smith, 1968*a*).

There is good evidence of low blood levels or tissue stores of vitamins amongst some old people living at home and in elderly patients in hospital. Such deficiency states were shown for thiamin by Griffiths *et al.* (1967), for folic acid by Hurdle & Picton-Williams (1966), for vitamin C by Andrews, Brook & Allen (1966) and by Milne *et al.* (1971) and for vitamin D by Exton-Smith, Hodkinson & Stanton (1966). The important question arises whether these low levels are abnormal and lead to the production of physical signs.

The authors quoted suggest that levels are abnormal because they can be raised by appropriate supplementation. Moreover, Brocklehurst and others (1968) reported improvement of physical signs on long-term supplementation with a multi-vitamin preparation. Later Dymock & Brocklehurst (1972) repeated the study on 126 old people in hospital of whom 77 survived the one year period of the clinical trial and were included in the analysis. Single vitamin supplementation was used and clinical improvement was noted as follows: (a) Riboflavin therapy was associated with an improvement in chielosis ($P<0.05$) and possible angular stomatitis. (b) Nicotinamide produced an improvement in the appearance of the dorsum of the tongue ($P<0.05$). (c) Ascorbic acid produced a mean rise of 2 g in the haemoglobin level ($P<0.01$).

Dymock & Brocklehurst (1972) concluded that old people with low vitamin levels may at least be in the process of developing physical changes. Biochemical indices of depletion of some members of the vitamin B complex are not yet sufficiently sensitive and the true correlations between biochemical depletion, physical signs and improvement on therapy have not yet been established. In view of the impaired homeostasis in old age the recognition of these preventible disorders is clearly important, especially as they can all be readily reversed by appropriate treatment.

Some nutritional deficiencies

The results of the Nutrition Survey of the Elderly (Department of Health and Social Security, 1972), based on random samples of old people living at home in six areas of the United Kingdom, show that malnutrition occurs in about 3 per cent of the elderly population. This includes protein energy malnutrition, iron deficiency and several vitamin deficiencies. In the majority of cases it was a direct consequence of physical or mental disorder. Nevertheless, environmental causes related to mode of living and other socio-economic factors may be of importance. Thus in the absence of overt malnutrition it was found that men over the age of 75 living alone fared worse than those living with a relative or spouse in respect of a large number of nutrients, and this was in some measure reflected in the proportion having biochemical levels below certain arbitrary limits; for example, four times as many men over 75 years of age living alone had leucocyte ascorbic acid levels below 7 $\mu g/10^8$ wbc compared with those living in the company of others. Similarly, both for men and women, there was a statistically significant higher incidence of anaemia in those living alone compared with that found in other groups.

Detection of malnutrition

The clinical significance of malnutrition is far greater than its incidence might suggest, since in almost every case it is treatable with excellent results. Difficulties in detection of the early signs of malnutrition are similar to those encountered in the early recognition of many disease in old age. But in the case of nutritional deficiencies there are two further difficulties; for almost every nutrient there is a long latent period before a low intake leads to overt clinical manifestations and early diagnosis must depend upon the finding of abnormalities in special tests, including biochemical and haematological investigations; secondly, in the elderly the true significance of departures from normality revealed by these tests is unknown. Many of the abnormalities can be related to low intakes of certain nutrients, but in old age there is considerable variation between individuals. Some of these problems are discussed in greater detail in the following sections dealing with vitamin C and vitamin D deficiencies. In general, however, it should be remembered that in younger persons the margin of safety is wide, but in old age homeostatic mechanisms are often impaired and the precarious physiological balance may be upset by the operation of medical and environmental hazards to which the elderly are prone. Frank malnutrition may be precipitated by such stress in those individuals whose nutrition is only marginally adequate (Exton-Smith, 1968*b*).

Vitamin C deficiency

The role of vitamin C in the prevention of scurvy has been known for more than two centuries and scurvy is now a rare disease. Occasional cases, however, are found amongst the elderly especially in men. The manifestations include weakness, anaemia, swelling and bleeding of the gums, 'sheet' haemorrhages in the skin of the arms and legs, and sometimes haemorrhages at other sites. Sublingual 'petechiae' have been regarded as an early sign of vitamin C deficiency, but Andrews, Letcher & Brook (1969) have shown by histological examination that these lesions are not haemorrhages but small aneurysmal dilatations of the minute vessels under the tongue. They do not disappear when the vitamin C intake is increased and it is unlikely therefore that they are due to acute vitamin C deficiency.

Although overt manifestations of scurvy are uncommon, the bodily stores of the vitamin C in many old people are low. Thus, low levels of leucocyte ascorbic acid have been reported by several observers; the levels are lower in the elderly than in younger subjects (Brook & Grimshaw, 1968), and lower in winter than in summer (Allen, Andrews & Brook, 1967). Milne and his colleagues (1971) measured the leucocyte ascorbic acid (LAA) levels and the vitamin C intakes in a random sample of 204 men and 247 women aged 62-94 years living in Edinburgh. The LAA mean values for women (23.88 $\mu g/10^8$ cells) were found to be significantly higher than for men (19.11 $\mu g/10^8$ cells). The values decreased with increasing age in women but not in men. They were significantly higher in both sexes in the six months July to December. Slightly more than half the subjects had intakes of less than 30 mg daily, 23.6 per cent of men and 28.1 per cent of women had intakes of less than 20 mg daily and 4.7 per cent of men and 3 per cent of women intakes less than 10 mg daily. A significantly greater proportion of both men and women had mean intakes of less than 30 mg daily in the months October to March compared with the months April to September. A moderate correlation was present between vitamin C intake and LAA level. It was also found that LAA levels increase in parallel with, but lag behind, seasonal increases in vitamin C intakes.

The Edinburgh study and other dietary surveys disclose that there are an appreciable number of old people who have an intake of less than 10 mg daily, which is known to be the amount required to prevent or cure scurvy (Bartley, Krebs & O'Brien, 1953). A high proportion of the elderly population are consuming less than the recommended allowance of 30 mg per day (Department of Health and Social Security, 1969). This allowance takes into account the changes in requirements due to stress and considerable individual variations in requirements which are known to exist (Srikantia, Mohanram & Krishnaswamy, 1970). The majority of people will not suffer from any ill-effects from a vitamin C intake of less than 30 mg, but our assessment is handicapped through lack of information of the levels of LAA required for the maintenance of health. A contribution to our knowledge has been provided by the work of Windsor & Williams (1970) who measured the total hydroxyproline excretion (THP) in the urine of elderly subjects with differing vitamin C status. THP is a measure of collagen metabolism and vitamin C is required for collagen synthesis. It was found that in old people with LAA levels of less than 15 $\mu g/10^8$ wbc the administration of vitamin C produced a rise in THP excretion whereas this did not occur when the LAA content was greater than 15 $\mu g/10^8$ wbc. It is reasonable to suppose that subclinical or clinical deficiency exists in people with LAA levels of less than 15 $\mu g/10^8$ wbc and there is evidence from studies in which this parameter has been measured that levels below this lower limit are commonly found in old people.

Longitudinal studies are required to establish the relationship between health and nutrition in old age. Hodkinson & Exton-Smith (1976) have reported the results of an investigation of the mortality in a five-year follow-up study of the participants in the 1967/68 DHSS nutrition survey. Nutritional factors which were significant in predicting mortality were found to be low vitamin C intake in men ($P<0.02$) and a low serum pyridoxine level in women ($P<0.01$). These findings must be interpreted with caution and further confirmatory studies are required to ascertain whether they represent true vitamin deficiencies. Another investigation has shown that leucocyte ascorbic acid level is a predictor of mortality in patients admitted to a geriatric department, but this was subsequently found to be an effect related to severity of illness and not an expression of deficiency of vitamin C since supplementation had no influence on survival (Wilson *et al.*, 1973). It is possible that the relationship between vitamin C intake and mortality is an epiphenomenon in that the fittest men may select diets which are particularly rich in vitamin C.

Vitamin D deficiency

Deficiency of vitamin D, producing osteomalacia, may be the result of several causes. The following are important factors in old age:

Dietary deficiency

Inadequate exposure to sunlight
Malabsorption syndromes (including postgastrectomy states, gluten enteropathy and possibly small-bowel ischaemia)
Liver and biliary tract disease
Renal disease

Several of these factors sometimes operate together; thus osteomalacia may appear in an old person who has mild degrees of malabsorption and who is housebound with a low dietary intake. At present the majority of cases of vitamin D deficiency are only recognised at an advanced stage when there are the typical biochemical findings or bone changes of osteomalacia. In his chapter Nordin shows that vitamin D lack may further impair the calcium absorption which is often already reduced in old age and this in turn may be responsible for osteoporosis. Thus mild, continued vitamin D deficiency may account for the increased porosity of bone in old age and the liability to fracture especially in elderly women.

The occurrence of vitamin D deficiency due to low dietary intake was assessed in the first King Edward's Hospital Fund Survey (Exton-Smith & Stanton, 1965). Following the dietary investigations, three-quarters of the elderly women agreed to participate in further studies involving clinical assessment, biochemical investigations and the determination of the radiographic density of bone (Exton-Smith *et al.*, 1966). Slightly more than one-quarter of the subjects were found to have marked skeletal rarefaction and when these subjects were compared with age-matched individuals whose bones were of higher density it was found that the former had significantly lower vitamin D intakes. Moreover, vitamin D intakes were correlated with alterations in the serum levels of calcium, inorganic phosphorus and alkaline phosphatase. Thus the findings of this study suggest that dietary vitamin D deficiency may contribute to the skeletal rarefaction which is so common in old age.

Smith & his colleagues (1964) assessed the vitamin D status of a group of women living in Michigan (average 60.6 years) and compared them with a group of women of similar age living in Puerto Rico. For the Michigan group the level of vitamin D in the blood (serum anti-rachitic activity) was significantly lower in those subjects with low bone density compared with those having normal bones and the level showed marked seasonal variation. By contrast, in Puerto Rico, where there is much greater exposure to sunlight and a higher vitamin D content of the food, the incidence of skeletal rarefaction was much lower, the serum vitamin D levels were much higher and there was no seasonal variation. The authors attributed the skeletal rarefaction to osteoporosis, rather than to osteomalacia, but they noted a correlation between the vitamin D levels and serum calcium, inorganic phosphorus and alkaline phosphatase.

Using the more precise index of radio-stereo-assay of 25 hydroxycholecalciferol levels, Stamp & Round (1974) have shown similar seasonal variations in both young and old subjects. They conclude that summer sunlight is an important, and possibly the chief, determinant of vitamin D nutrition in Britain. In this study, the older people who participated in a nutrition survey in the London Borough of Camden, had significantly lower levels of 25 hydroxycholecalciferol than those found in the younger subjects.

Clinical osteomalacia may not be rare in certain sections of the elderly population. Thus Anderson & his colleagues (1966) in Glasgow found 16 cases after thorough investigation of 100 women admitted to a geriatric department and who had a possible clinical indication, namely, vague and generalised pain, bone tenderness, low backache, muscle weakness and stiffness, waddling gait, skeletal deformity, malabsorption states, long confinement indoors or malnutrition. Subsequently 100 consecutive admissions to the female geriatric wards were investigated and the incidence of osteomalacia was found to be 4 per cent of all elderly women. The authors considered the osteomalacia to be due mainly to dietary lack of vitamin D and to insufficient synthesis in the skin due to inadequate exposure to sunlight.

The importance of vitamin D deficiency in the causation of fractures and other orthopaedic problems in the elderly has been recognised by Chalmers & his colleagues (1967). They have described the clinical features of 37 patients with osteomalacia and the majority were elderly women. They emphasize the need for thorough screening of all elderly patients presenting with weakness, skeletal pain, pathological fractures, or with diminished radiographic density of bone. They attributed the osteomalacia to dietary deficiency of vitamin D, inadequate exposure to sunlight and mild degrees of malabsorption occurring alone or in combination.

The difficulties inherent in the detection of vitamin D deficiency in old age are immense and these problems have been discussed elsewhere (Exton-Smith 1968*b*). It is clearly desirable to look more diligently for cases of osteomalacia amongst the elderly population and undoubtedly many cases of dietary origin will be discovered. The importance lies in the fact that the condition is so readily preventible by increased vitamin D intake and the disease when it is recognised responds most satisfactorily to treatment. Particular attention must be paid to the housebound who probably represent the largest single vulnerable group. A study of housebound old people (Exton-Smith, Stanton & Windsor, 1972) disclosed that 48 per cent of housebound women aged 70-79 years have a vitamin D intake of less than 30iu per day, compared with 13 per cent of active women of similar age. For those confined to the house, lack of exposure to sunlight is a significant additional factor.

The question has arisen whether vitamin D deficiency is of clinical importance in the absence of the usual features of osteomalacia. Aaron and her colleagues (1974*a*) in Leeds have shown by histological methods that 20 to 30 per cent of women with fracture of the proximal femur and about 40 per cent of men had osteomalacia. Later they showed (Aaron, Gallagher & Nordin, 1974*b*) that the proportion with osteomalacia varied with the season. The highest frequency of abnormal calcification fronts (43 per cent) was observed in February to April and the lowest (15 per cent) in August to October. The highest frequency of abnormal osteoid covered surfaces (47 per cent) was observed in April to June and the lowest (13 per cent) in October to December. They concluded that variation in hours of sunshine is responsible for a seasonal variation in osteomalacia in femoral neck fractures and, possibly, in the elderly population as a whole. The significane of vitamin D deficiency as an important factor in the pathogenesis of fracture of the femoral neck has been confimed by the study of Faccini, Exton-Smith & Boyde (1976). The mean value of trabecular osteoid area in the fracture group was 4 per cent compared with 1 per cent in a control group. The difference was also striking in the proportion of trabecular surface covered by osteoid; the mean value for the fracture group was 24.5 per cent compared with 7.9 per cent for the control group. Brown, Bakowska & Millard (1976) found significantly lower levels of 25 hydroxycholecalciferol in patients with fracture of the femoral neck compared with those in controls of similar age from whom blood samples were taken at the same time of year. This is believed to be a reflection of the decreased out-of-doors activity of the patients prior to their fracture.

Prevention of malnutrition

In order to be able to prevent malnutrition in old people, not only do we need information on dietary intakes, their state of health and their special nutritional requirements, but also an understanding of their way of life and the reasons why inadequate intakes occur. The results of the survey carried out by the Department of Health and Social Security (1972) in six centres in Great Britain showed a small incidence of frank malnutrition; nevertheless a proportion of the elderly had very low intakes of certain nutrients and under the stress of adverse circumstances subnutrition might develop. Unless these vulnerable groups can be recognised, preventative measures would have to be applied to all, even though the vast majority will never suffer from malnutrition. The inefficiency of such procedures can only be overcome by the identification of those especially at risk; the application of preventative measures to these smaller groups rather than to the whole elderly population is a manageable preposition. It is believed that the housebound form the largest single group at risk (Exton-Smith *et al.*, 1972). The prevention of malnutrition in this group should present less difficulty than that in other vulnerable groups which cannot be so readily identified since the majority of housebound old people are known to the health and social services.

Recognition of early signs

The difficulties of detection of the early signs of malnutrition are similar to those encountered in the early recognition of many diseases in old age. Williamson & his colleagues (1964) investigated all patients over the age of 65 on the lists of three general practitioners and found that men had a mean of 3.26 disabilities of which 1.87 were unknown to the general practitioners and women a mean of 3.42 disabilities of which 2.03 were unknown. It can be concluded from this and other studies that many old people do not report their complaints to doctors until the condition is advanced. Thus a service based on the self-reporting of illness is likely to be severely handicapped in meeting the needs of old people. Williamson & co-workers (1964) emphasized that preventive medicine is at least as important in old age as it is in earlier life since in old people there are few conditions that medical and social measures applied soon enough will not help. These considerations apply equally to nutritional disorders, which are so readily preventible, or should be treated promptly once they have occurred.

Several means have been suggested for overcoming the handicap arising from lack of reporting of illness by old people (Exton-Smith, 1968*a*) and a method which is offering promise of success is the use of health visitors (or geriatric visitors) for the first tier of the screening. They act on behalf of those who are thought to be especially at risk on general practitioners' lists. Thus priority in visiting is given to the recently bereaved, the socially isolated, the housebound, and those old people, who according to the general practitioners' records, have not consulted their doctor during the previous 12 months. Voluntary bodies such as local old people's welfare committees can play a useful role by compiling and keeping up-to-date lists of people in the vulnerable groups and arranging for regular visits by voluntary workers. By these means it is hoped that the early signs of medical and social breakdown will be detected.

The assessment of dietary intakes should ideally be made by dietitians, but their skills are rarely available for old people at home. Simple scoring systems based on the number of main meals and the frequency of consumption of certain foods containing protein (meat, cheese, eggs, bread and milk) have been devised and these can readily be applied by a health visitor to give a rough guide on the quality of the diet (Marr, Heady & Morris, 1961).

Club meals and meals-on-wheels

It has been shown that nutrient intakes often improve when old people eat at clubs in the company of others. Many old people find it is more convenient to have a club meal since there is no shopping, food preparation or washing-up to be done. The King Edward's Hospital Fund Survey (1965) showed that in order to make an effective contribution to the total dietary intake at least four club meals a week should be eaten. The survey revealed a considerable variation in the quality and amount of food served. In the best centre surveyed the five meals a week which were served provided over one-third of the total nutrient intake. The club meal must be as nutritious as possible since the recipient tends to regard it as the main meal of the day and often takes only snacks at other times.

About 1.5 per cent of old people receive domiciliary meals (Department of Health and Social Security, 1970). There is need for a considerable expansion of this service, since Townsend & Wedderburn (1965) discovered that another 5 per cent would like to receive meals. The meals service is usually provided by the WRVS and the regular visits to the homes of housebound old people does much to prevent social isolation. Probably the main disadvantage of the present system is that the meal must be cooked and kept warm for several hours before it reaches the patient's home. By this time the meal may appear unattractive and at least some of its nutritive value will have been lost. The loss of vitamin C, for example, during the time the meal is cooked and kept hot can be as much as 90 per cent.

There is need for experiment in this field. In several areas the provision of frozen meals has been tried. A supply of food is delivered only once a week, thus the service is economical in personnel and the meal can be cooked immediately before it is eaten. The main disadvantages, however, are that there may be no proper facilities for storage, the patient may be unable to cook the meal himself by reason of physical or mental incapacity and he is visited much less frequently by voluntary workers.

Food education

To remedy the ignorance about food which is common amongst old people, instruction can be given by dietitians or health visitors. In many cases to be effective this instruction has to be given individually, but this is time-consuming. Moreover, the necessary skills are not available, so individual instruction should be reserved mainly for those people in the vulnerable groups. For active old people, cookery classes are proving popular and they help to promote good nutrition. Sometimes these classes are organised by Education Authorities and the old people who attend register as students. Not only do they learn about cooking but in some cases their interest is so enlivened that they register for classes in other subjects as well.

At present many old people living alone are handicapped by the difficulty in finding small portions of nutritious but readily prepared food. Thus they tend to select those items which require little preparation and are often of low nutritive value. The food industry could make an important contribution by studying the needs of single old people and marketing suitable foods.

Supplementation

The most satisfactory means of improving the nutrition of old people is by improving the quality, and in some cases the quantity, of their diet. The very low intakes of certain nutrients (for example, vitamin C and vitamin D) especially amongst the vulnerable groups must lead to consideration of the possibility of supplementation. In the nutrition survey of the housebound (Exton-Smith *et al.*, 1972) it was found that 12 per cent had vitamin C intakes of less than 10mg per day which is the amount required for the prevention or cure of scurvy. When dietary assessment reveals very low consumption of vitamin C, intake should be improved by the addition to the diet of citrus fruit, blackcurrant juice, rose-hip syrup or tomatoes. The alternative method of increasing intake by prescription of vitamin C tablets is satisfactory, but less desirable.

The same survey of the housebound revealed that low vitamin D intakes are common; furthermore, in those confined to the house, lack of exposure to sunlight leads to deficient synthesis of vitamin D in the skin. Although the precise requirements are unknown the housebound were found to have a statistically significant difference in their vitamin D intakes compared with the general elderly population. It must be emphasized, however, that according to the National Food Surveys, the mean intakes of the elderly in general are similar to those of the younger population. A means of increasing intake would be by the fortification of milk which is a procedure used in the US. There is believed to be considerable individual variation in vitamin D requirements and since in some persons moderately excessive intakes can lead to vitamin D intoxication, the distribution of fortified milk would best be restricted to vulnerable groups such as the housebound.

It is important that policy of supplementation should only be decided after the results of carefully controlled experiments are available to assess the benefit derived from increased intakes. Once supplementation is introduced and becomes widespread it is difficult to prove or assess the benefits. Moreover there is an understandable reluctance to withdraw a preventive measure on the basis of doubts about its value when it has been practised for a number of years.

Department of Health and Social Security: 'Nutrition and health in old age'
The DHSS has recently published a report *(Nutrition and health in old age,* Reports on Health and Social Subjects No. 16, 1979. London: HMSO) based on a cross-sectional analysis of the findings derived from examination of 365 old people who participated in surveys in 1967/68 and in 1972/73.

In the second survey 26 per cent of the subjects who were all over the age of 70 years were judged on clinical grounds to be suffering from malnutrition. For those aged 70-80 years the prevalence was 6 per cent for men and 5 per cent for women, but for those aged 80 years and over the rates had almost doubled to 12 per cent for men and 8 per cent for women. The types of malnutrition included protein energy, iron, vitamin B group, folate, ascorbic acid and vitamin D deficiencies. Several subjects had evidence of multiple nutrient deficiencies. Both men and women over 80 years of age who were malnourished had mean daily intakes of animal protein, vitamin C and vitamin D which were significantly lower ($P<0.01$) than the expected mean intakes, and men over 80 years old had a significantly lower intake of nicotinic acid. Thus the diets of the malnourished were generally poor in quality. Eleven risk factors associated with malnutrition were identified and these were: living alone, no regular cooked meals, receipt of supplementary benefit, social classes IV and V, a low mental test score, depression, chronic bronchitis and emphysema, partial gastrectomy, poor dentition, difficulty in swallowing and the housebound state. Malnutrition was significantly associated ($P<0.001$) with the occurrence of multiple risk factors. The housebound who constituted 12.6 per cent of all the survey subjects were found to be an important and readily identifiable group at risk of malnutrition. Of the malnourished subjects 31 per cent were completely housebound compared with 11 per cent of the non-malnourished subjects. Housebound men have lower mean dietary intakes of protein, iron and riboflavine than the non-housebound men and housebound women had significantly lower mean intakes of food energy, iron, riboflavine and ascorbic acid than the non-housebound women. In general, elderly malnourished people in the United Kingdom have individual problems which require the personal attention of general practitioners, health visitors, social workers and where possible, relatives and friends.

For the prevention of malnutrition in old age particular attention should be paid to the following points. Those who are housebound and, therefore, have little exposure to sunlight, can develop osteomalacia; few foods contain any vitamin D but the deficiency can be prevented or corrected by giving supplements. Those who have had a partial gastrectomy often develop anaemia and evidence of other nutrient deficiencies. Those who are unable to cope because of mental or physical disability may also develop generalised malnutrition or particular deficiency diseases such as scurvy, especially when they live alone. These deficiencies can be easily corrected by a better quality diet or by the necessary supplement. Much can be done to improve nutritional status of those who live alone, have been bereaved or are depressed, if they can be encouraged to overcome their loneliness and make use of the facilities for meals at clubs and day centres or increase their contact with friends and relatives.

References

Aaron, J.E. Gallagher, J.C., Anderson, J., Stasiak, L., Longton, E.B., Nordin, B.E.C. & Nicholson, M. (1974*a*): *Lancet* 1, 229.

Aaron, J.E., Gallagher, J.C. & Nordin, B.E.C. (1974*b*): *Lancet* 2, 84.

Allen, M.A., Andrews, J. & Brook, M. (1967): *Nutr. Diet.* 21, 136.

Allen, T.H., Anderson, E.C. & Langham, W.H. (1960): *J. Geront.* 15, 348.

Anderson, I., Campbell, A.E.R., Dunn, A. & Runciman, J.B.M. (1966): *Scot. Med. J.* 11, 429.

Anderson, W.F. (1967): *Practical management of the elderly.* Oxford: Blackwell.

Andrews, J., Letcher, M. & Brook, M. (1969): *Br. Med. J.* 2, 415.

Andrews, J., Brook, M. & Allen, M.A. (1966): *Geront. Clin. (Basel).* 8, 257.

Bartley, W., Krebs, H.A. & O'Brien, J.R.P. (1953): *Vitamin C requirements of human adults.* Spec. Rep. Ser. Med. Res. Counc. No. 280. London: HMSO.

Brockington, F. & Lempert, S.M. (1967): *The Stockport Survey. The social needs of the over 80s.* Manchester: University Press.

Brocklehurst, J., Griffiths, L.L., Taylor, G.F., Marks, J. & Scott, D.L. (1968): *Geront. Clin. (Basel).* 10, 309.

Brook, M. & Grimshaw, J.J. (1968): *Am. J. Clin. Nutr.* 21, 1254.

Brown, I.R.F., Bakowska, A. & Millard, P.H. (1976): *Age & Ageing* 5, 127.

Chalmers, J., Conacher, W.D.H., Gardner, D.L. & Scott, P.J. (1967): *J. Bone. Jt Surg.* **49B**, 403.

Chope, H.D. & Breslow, L. (1956): *Am. J. Publ. Hlth* **46**, 61.

Department of Health and Social Security (1969): *Recommended intakes of nutrients for the United Kingdom.* Rep. Publ. Hlth Med. Subj. No. 120. London: HMSO.

Department of Health and Social Security (1970): *First report by the Panel on Nutrition of the Elderly.* Rep. Publ. Hlth Med. Subj. No. 123. London: HMSO.

Department of Health and Social Security (1972): *A nutrition survey of the elderly.* London: HMSO.

Dymock, S. & Brocklehurst, J. (1972): Paper given at meeting of British Geriatrics Society, London.

Exton-Smith, A.N. (1968*a*): *Roy. Soc. Hlth J.* **88**, 205.

Exton-Smith, A.N. (1968*b*): In *Vitamins in the elderly,* ed A.N. Exton-Smith & D.L. Scott. Bristol: Wright.

Exton-Smith, A.N. (1970): *Nutrition, Lond.* 24, 218.

Exton-Smith, A.N. & Stanton, B.R. (1965): An investigation of the dietary of elderly women living alone. London: King Edward's Hospital Fund.

Exton-Smith, A.N., Hodkinson, H.M. & Stanton, B.R. (1966): *Lancet* 2, 999.

Exton-Smith, A.N., Stanton, B.R. & Windsor, A.C.M. (1972): *Nutrition of housebound old people.* London: King Edward's Hospital Fund.

Faccini, J.M., Exton-Smith, A.N. & Boyde, A. (1976): *Lancet* 1, 1089.

Fowlie, H.C., Cohen, C. & Anand, M.P. (1963): *Geront. Clin. (Basel)* 5, 215.

Gillum, H.L. & Morgan, A.F. (1955): *J. Nutr.* 55, 265.

Griffiths, L.L., Brocklehurst, J.C., Scott, D.L., Marks, J. & Blackley, J. (1967): *Geront. Clin. (Basel)* 9, 1.

Hodkinson, H.M. & Exton-Smith, A.N. (1976): *Age & Ageing* 5, 110.

Hurdle, A.D. & Williams, T.C.P. (1966): *Br. Med. J.* 2, 202.

Marr, J., Heady, J.A. & Morris, J. (1961): Proc. 3rd Int. Congress Dietetics, London.

Milne, J.S., Lonergan, M.E., Williamson, J., Moore, F.M.L., McMaster, R. & Percy, N. (1971): *Br. Med. J.* 4, 383.

Sheldon, J.H. (1948): *The social medicine of old age.* London: Oxford University Press.

Smith, R.W., Rizek, J., Frame, B. & Mansour, J. (1964): *Am. J. Clin. Nutr.* **14**, 98.

Srikantia, S.G., Mohanram, M. & Krishnaswamy, K. (1970): *Am. J. Clin. Nutr.* 23, 59.

Stamp, T.C.B. & Round, J.M. (1974): *Nature,* **247**, 563.

Stanton, B.R. & Exton-Smith, A.N. (1970): *A longitudinal study of the dietary of elderly women.* London: King Edward's Hospital Fund.

Steinkamp, R.C., Cohen, N.L. & Walsh, H.E. (1965): *J.Am. Diet. Ass.* **46**, 103.

Stokoe, I.H. (1965): Psychiatric disorders of the aged. Report on the Symposium held by the World Psychiatric Association, London.

Townsend, P. & Wedderburn, D. (1965): *The aged in the welfare state.* London: Bell & Sons.
Watkin, D.M. (1968): In *Vitamins in the elderly,* ed A.N. Exton-Smith & D.L. Scott. Bristol: Wright.
Williamson, J. *et al.* (1964): *Lancet* 1, 1117.
Wilson, T.S., Datta, S.B., Murrell, J.S. & Andrews, C.T. (1973): *Age & Ageing* 2, 163.
Windsor, A.C.M. & Williams, C.B. (1970): *Br. Med. J.* 1, 731.

10

Assessing the nutritional status of the population

Sylvia J. Darke.

Introduction

Malnutrition has been defined as any disturbance of form or function of the body which is due to either a deficiency or an excess of one or more essential nutrients or to an imbalance of nutrients, that is to say, a relative excess of some nutrients with a deficiency of others. Thus, to be of good nutritional status a person must be free from the diseases of malnutrition. Nutritional status is inevitably bound up with health and well-being, but just as there is no easy way to measure health, there is also no simple or single measurement upon which an assessment of nutritional status can be made. Information must be gathered from a number of different sources.

A first essential for good nutritional status is access to enough of a mixture of different foods, since only the young infant from birth up to about six months can rely on a single food (human milk) as the sole source of essential nutrients. In older individuals, providing energy requirements are met by food intake and the diet includes a mixture of foods, the body selects the different nutrients in the amounts required. Thus, if the requirements of each individual for energy and for nutrients were known, a diet which supplied these requirements (no more and no less) would ensure a satisfactory nutritional status. But, for most nutrients, requirements are not known and vary from one individual to another even when individuals are of the same age, sex and size, and carry out the same activities. Thus information about food eaten cannot in practice measure nutritional status, although such information can be useful in identifying different types of malnutrition. To ensure adequate food supplies goes a long way towards maintaining good health, and information about food supplies and food intake is therefore of some, but limited, value in assessing nutritional status.

Government is concerned with the nutritional status of the whole population and with food and nutrition policy. Food policy should ensure the provision of safe, wholesome food, which is palatable and in sufficient amount to meet demand. A nutrition policy, on the other hand, is concerned with the nutrient quality of the diet and with ensuring that all sections of the population can procure enough of a mixture of foods for health. If such policies are to be effective in maintaining the health of the nation they must be based on sound nutritional and economic evidence. Assessment of nutritional status thus becomes a matter of some importance. In addition, because nutritional effects may reveal themselves either in the short or long term, the collection of information should be a continuous process.

Indicators of nutritional status

The so-called 'running indices' of nutrition are potential sources of information about nutritional status. They are statistics collected on a regular basis by different government departments and provide information either about food supplies or different aspects of health.

Food supply statistics and their use

(a) Consumption level estimates (CLE). Information about food supplies in the United Kingdom is published annually by the Ministry of Agriculture, Fisheries and Food and is of two kinds. The first is basic information about the total amount of food produced annually in this country minus the amount exported together with the amount imported, that is to say, the total amount of food available at the farm gate and dock side. Table 1 shows food supply statistics for 1958, 1968 and 1978 expressed as available food energy and nutrients per head of the population per day.

Table 1. Total supplies of energy and of some nutrients from food (excluding alcohol) in the United Kingdom/person/day: according to Ministry of Agriculture, Fisheries and Food 'Food facts' 1973 and 1979

		1958	1968	1978
Energy	kcal	3180	3090	2920
	MJ	13.3	12.9	12.2
Animal protein	g	49.1	52.5	51.4
Vegetable protein	g	34.3	32.8	31.4
Total protein	g	83.4	85.3	82.8
Fat	g	141	144	130
Carbohydrate	g	423	387	379
Calcium	mg	1130	1130	1080
Iron	mg	15.5	14.8	13.1
Vitamin A	iu	4460	4750	4567
Retinol equiv	μg	–	–	1370
Thiamin	mg	1.74	1.84	1.68
Riboflavin	mg	1.83	1.98	1.92
Total niacin	mg	16.6	18.7	19.7
Niacin equiv	mg	–	–	34.3
Vitamin C	mg	95	104	102
Vitamin D	μg	3.70	1.34	2.73

Food energy supplies have decreased slightly in response to a falling demand which reflects a life style that depends on labour-saving devices in the home and factory and relies upon the motorcar and television for leisure activities. Nutrient supplies have also varied slightly over the 20 years.

(b) National Food Survey (NFS). The Ministry also publishes annually the results of the National Food Survey. This survey, which is unique to Great Britain, records continuously, except during the Christmas period, for a sample of some 7500 households each year, the amounts and cost of food purchased for domestic 'consumption' that is to say, household use over a period of one week. Allowance is made for the fact that some members of the family have some meals away from home, for food which is home grown or received as a gift, and for wastage. Certain foods – alcohol, sweets and soft drinks – are not included. The figures (averages for households) are expressed as weights of foods per head per week and as total food energy and nutrients per head per day. The NFS began in 1940 when the government needed to monitor food supplies to poor families in urban districts, but since 1950 the sample has included families in all income groups and from both rural and urban areas. The sample is stratified by region of the country, family size and income of the head of the household. The response rate is low (55-60 per cent), as might be expected when a great deal of information is required from a housewife on a purely voluntary basis. The survey provides useful information about trends in domestic food purchases, and although such 'consumption' figures do not necessarily equate with, they relate to, food actually eaten.

Table 2 shows food bought by the average household in 1958, 1968 and 1978 expressed as energy and nutrients per person per day. The difference between figures from the NFS and consumption level estimates is largely explained by the wastage of supplies during distribution to the retailer, and because the latter survey

Table 2. Food obtained for domestic use expressed as energy and nutrients/person/day and as a percentage of the current recommendation (Ministry of Agriculture, Fisheries and Foods 1960, 1970, 1979; British Medical Association, 1950; Department of Health and Social Security, 1969)

		Energy and nutrients/ person/day			Energy and nutrients expressed as a percentage of the current recommendation			
		1958	1968	1978	1958 (BMA)	1968 (BMA)	1968 (DHSS)	1978 (DHSS)
Energy	kcal	2600	2560	2260	104	107	108	94
	MJ	–	10.7	9.5				
Animal protein	g	43.4	46.6	46.3				
Vegetable protein	g	31.2	28.7	26.3				
Total protein	g	74.6	75.4	72.6	100	106	127	121
Fat	g	111	118	106				
Carbohydrate	g	325	318	272				
Calcium	mg	1040	1040	990	107	111	191	181
Iron	mg	14.2	13.5	11.2	115	114	122	100
Vitamin A	iu	4350	4670	–	184			
Retinol equiv	μg	–	1400	1490	–	203	203	212
Thiamin	mg	1.25	1.29	1.19	126	136	133	125
Riboflavin	mg	1.64	1.81	1.95	108	125	129	138
Total niacin	mg	13.6	15.7	16.5	137	–	–	–
Niacin equiv	mg	–	29	29.5	–	166	189	188
Vitamin C	mg	49	52	54	222	247	181	188
Vitamin D	μg	3.33	3.14	2.65		90	90	83

includes food used in institutional and commercial catering. The figures are interesting in that they show the trends in food supplies. Using National Food Survey statistics, because they are closest to 'food eaten' the percentage of the total food energy available from protein was 11.5 per cent in 1958, 11.6 per cent in 1968 and 12.8 per cent in 1978; the percentage of energy from carbohydrate was 54 per cent in 1958, 50 per cent in 1968 and 48 per cent in 1978; that from fat was 38 per cent in 1958, 41 per cent in 1968 and 43 per cent in 1978 (Ministry of Agriculture, Fisheries and Food, 1960, 1970 and 1979).

In order to assess the adequacy of food supplies a comparison with some yardstick is necessary. The yardstick figures which are in general use are called 'Recommended allowances' (British Medical Association, 1950), 'Recommended intakes' (Department of Health and Social Security, 1969), and 'Recommended amounts of energy and the different nutrients' (Department of Health and Social Security, 1979). The figures are based on estimates of requirements from such experimental evidence as there is and include for most nutrients a wide safety margin. The figures refer only to groups of the population of the same sex, age and degree of physical activity. Thus, if the food available for the group is such that, on average, each individual could have the recommended amount for energy and the different nutrients, and if each ate only what they needed individuals would actually eat different amounts. About half would eat less and half more than the amount recommended, and the requirements of all individuals in the population would be covered. If, therefore, available food supplies meet the recommended amounts the assumption can be made that any risk of undernutrition is minimal and the possibility of good nutritional status is assured, except for those who elect to eat diets which are unusual either in quantity or quality.

Table 2 compares the energy and nutrient content of food purchased by the average household with the recommended amounts then currently in use and shows that, by and large, in Great Britain the available food supply was consistent with the amounts recommended to cover the needs of most of the population. The assessment is very inexact because, as has already been stressed, the figures for recommended amounts are approximations due to an insufficiency of accurate quantitative knowledge of individual requirements. Nevertheless the comparison is reassuring for the United Kingdom. Were a similar comparison possible in respect of countries described as belonging to 'the third world' the result might well be different.

The figures can be analysed according to different socio-economic groupings and, providing the sample is sufficiently large, statistics for groups within the population which are considered to be 'at-risk' of undernutrition can be examined separately. The average supply figure for members of large family households may be less than that recommended. This does not indicate undernutrition necessarily. All that can be inferred is that the smaller the average figure is compared with the recommended amount the greater the possibility of undernutrition in some individuals. To ascertain whether or not individuals are malnourished, in-depth nutritional surveys should be made in which individual food intakes are measured, and medical assessments, anthropometric measurements, biochemical and haematological examinations are included.

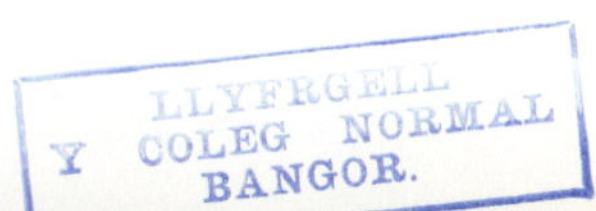

(c) Family Expenditure Survey. The Department of Employment has been responsible for the Family Expenditure Survey since it began in 1957 although sampling, field work and coding are done by the Office of Population Censuses and Surveys. In addition to expenditure on many other items, the survey provides information about the amount of money spent on food by the household per week and about money spent on different items of food. This information can be compared with that obtained from the National Food Survey statistics on food costs for the household for the week of the survey. Food costs are of significance in respect of ensuring the availability of enough food to all individuals. The survey also shows trends in the proportion of income spent on food.

Health statistics

Not all the health statistics which are collected have the same relative importance in the assessment of nutritional status. Nevertheless there are several different 'running indices' which need to be considered when deriving the composite picture.

(a) 'Vital statistics' provide information about birth and death and are supplied by the Office of Population Censuses and Surveys. Birth statistics include infant mortality, still birth, low birth weight, neonatal and perinatal mortality rates. Figure 1 shows a continued steady improvement in the national figures. The figures are periodically analysed by social class, and age and parity of the mother so that, although information about nutrition is not directly available, the statistics are useful because they reflect changes in the situation of a 'worst-off' minority.

In the same way, death rates can contribute to the overall picture of nutritional status for those diseases known or suspected to have a nutritional factor in

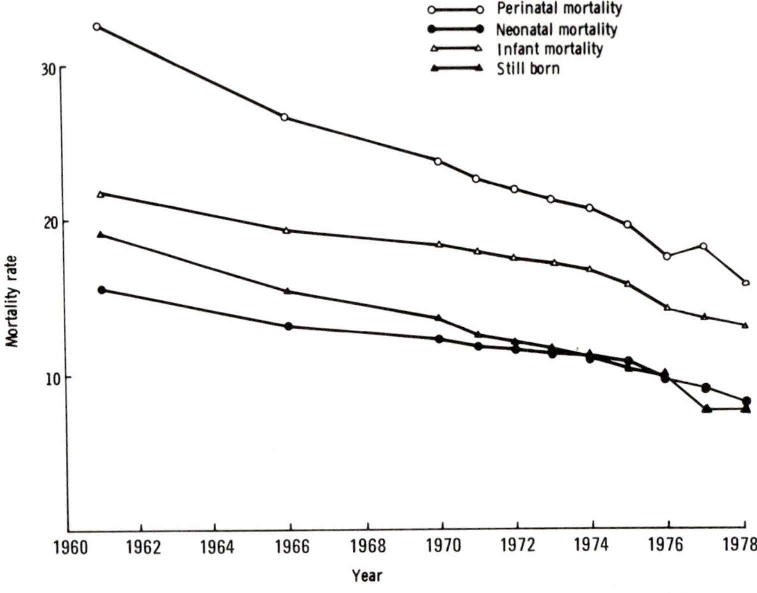

Fig. 1. Vital statistics (Great Britain) – Office of Population Censuses and Surveys (1975, 1978, 1979)

Table 3. Chronic sickness. Persons reporting long-standing illness by sex, age and socio-economic group: rates per 1000. (Office of Population Censuses and Surveys, 1977)

All persons **Great Britain**

	Males					Females				
Socio-economic group*	**Total**	0-14	15-44	45-64	**65+**	**Total**	0-14	15-44	45-64	65+
Professional	141	57	122	215	(24)†	154	46	149	309	(12)†
Employers and managers	185	96	141	230	417	176	61	133	211	524
Intermediate and junior non-manual	226	95	150	372	460	222	63	113	309	516
Skilled manual (incl. foremen and supervisors) and own account non-professional	202	97	140	317	508	198	81	159	285	518
Semi-skilled manual and personal service	222	79	154	332	492	280	51	160	354	575
Unskilled manual	308	89	210	500	456	314	81	140	350	532
Rate for all persons in each sex/age group	206	91	145	313	466	224	68	143	300	532

*See appendix A, pp. 187-8. Members of the Armed Forces, inadequately described occupations, and all persons (including students) who have never worked have not been shown as separate categories. They are, however, included in the rates for all persons.

†The number of observations only is shown in parentheses where the base figure is less than 100

the aetiology. Analysis of the figures by different socio-economic factors can help in assessing the condition of population groups which are 'at-risk' for one reason or another.

(b) The General Household Survey is the responsibility of the Office of Population Censuses and Surveys. It is an inter-departmental survey which began in 1971 and is sponsored by the Central Statistical Office. Information about self-reported chronic and acute ill-health is obtained from approximately 15 000 households annually in Great Britain. Table 3 gives figures for 'chronic sickness' according to age, sex and different socio-economic groups. As might be expected, longstanding illness is reported more frequently by the elderly and those in unskilled manual occupations. However, no direct assessment of the relative importance of nutritional factors is possible because codes for disease categories are too broad to determine whether or not nutrition is a factor.

(c) The Department of Health and Social Security publishes annually morbidity statistics from the hospital in-patient enquiry which provides information about diseases of under-and-over-nutrition seen in hospitals. The figures refer to 10 per cent of all hospital discharges and do not provide incidence statistics since the same individual may be discharged from two or more spells in hospital in any one year. The hospital activity analysis provide similar information for local areas. The information is useful in that trends in disease patterns with time can be seen. For example the incidence of rickets and osteomalacia – which occur in Asian children and young women – can be seen to have increased in the early 1960s when immigration was at its height, and from 1972/3 onwards to show a steady decline (Department of Health and Social Security, 1980 – to be published).

(d) Heights and weights of schoolchildren are measured during the routine medical examination at school entry and school leaving. The information is analysed centrally by the Scottish Home and Health Department, but not in England and Wales. Gradients in height and weight associated with family size, and socio-economic differences still persist. Children from small families and Registrar General social classes I and II on average grow to be taller and heavier compared with children from large families and Registrar General social classes IV and V (Tables 4 and 5). Genetic and environmental factors other than nutrition are important in these differences. The factors include the relationship and interaction between the child and the mother (of special importance immediately after birth and in early childhood), and with other members of the family, and the amount of stimulation which the child receives from the external environmental (Sosa *et al.*, 1976).

(e) The last of the 'running-indices' of nutrition are figures derived from the Blood Transfusion Service in England and Wales. Area directors make monthly returns to the Department of Health and Social Security of the numbers of new female volunteer blood donors of child-bearing age who are rejected because

Table 4. Mean heights and weights of school leavers from families of different sizes in Scotland* 1970/71†: Scottish Home and Health Department (Personal communication)

No. in Family	Boys Mean ht (in)	Boys Mean wt (lb)	Girls Mean ht (in)	Girls Mean wt (lb)
1	61.3	103.4	61.3	108.1
2	61.2	100.8	61.3	100.7
3	60.7	98.0	61.0	104.6
4	60.4	96.3	60.6	102.6
5	60.0	94.5	60.2	100.6
6	59.7	93.9	60.0	99.8
7+	59.4	92.5	59.5	97.6

*Excluding Aberdeen City and Aberdeen County
†10 per cent sample of records

Table 5. Mean heights and weights of school leavers from families of different social class in Scotland,* 1970/71†; Scottish Home and Health Department (Personal communication)

Social class	Boys Mean ht (in)	Boys Mean wt (lb)	Girls Mean ht (in)	Girls Mean wt (lb)
1	61.8	101.8	61.4	103.3
2	61.5	102.2	61.2	106.1
3	60.5	97.2	60.7	103.0
4	60.2	95.4	60.5	102.6
5	59.6	94.3	59.7	100.7

*Excluding Aberdeen City and Aberdeen County
†10 per cent sample of records

their haemoglobin is below the accepted standard. The figures give some assessment, albeit very approximate, of anaemia in a self-selected sample of women of child-bearing age.

Assessment of nutritional status by nutrition surveys

'Nutrition surveys' have been made by the Department of Health and Social Security (DHSS), by academic departments of universities and medical schools and by research groups under the aegis of the Medical Research Council.

Surveys made by the DHSS in the past decade are listed in Table 6. A pilot study of 435 pre-schoolchildren in 1963 (Ministry of Health, 1968) tested the feasibility of the field methods, the use of the Food Composition Tables‡ (specially prepared and continually updated for later surveys), and of processing and analysis of results by computer (which at that time was a comparatively new tool for survey work). In contrast to some other countries, notably Canada and the United States of America, in which all age and sex groups were investigated in a single survey, the Department has made separate studies of individuals of different ages.

Samples were randomly selected and were of people living in their own homes

‡*Copies on application from: Mrs M.M. Disselduff, Department of Health and Social security, London SE1 6BY.*

not in institutions. Areas were chosen both because a nutritional problem was thought to exist there and because local specialists within the National Health Service were willing to co-operate. Samples were usually biassed in favour of those sections of the population who were more likely to be at risk of malnutrition. The nutrition surveys have included preschoolchildren, schoolchildren, of pre- or early puberty (aged 10-11 years), adolescents aged 14-15 years, a comparatively small sample of children from one parent families, and a study of pregnant women. All these studies were cross-sectional in design.

Studies of the elderly have been both cross-sectional and longitudinal. The 1967/68 sample of elderly people over the age of 65 years were re-surveyed in 1972/73. All but three of the 879 participants in 1967/68 were traced, 277 were dead and 483 participated in the second study. The field work of the ten-year follow-up study of the 1967/68 cohort was completed by the end of 1978. The 1973/74 study of the elderly was a larger sample (some 1400), nationally representative and planned to be the first of a series of longitudinal studies which would provide continued surveillance of the elderly in the population.

Participation in all the studies was voluntary and included the completion of a socio-economic questionnaire by the dietary investigator, and a weighed record of all food and drink, including school meals, consumed over a period of seven consecutive days. Because information about dietary intake cannot itself be diagnostic of nutritional status, all survey subjects had a medical assessment and measurements of height and weight and skinfold thickness at various sites. In addition blood was taken from the elderly subjects for biochemistry and haematology, and radiology of both hands was included.

Results of the surveys. Among all the children surveyed a medical examination revealed no clinical signs of nutritional deficiency. The subjective medical assessment of nutritional status was based on the criteria set out in the International Biological Programme (IBP) handbook (Weiner & Laurie, 1969), and the vast majority of children were categorised as of 'good' nutritional status, 1-4 per cent in the different surveys as of 'average' nutritional status, and none as of 'poor' status. By contrast 4-8 per cent of the children were assessed as obese (Department of Health and Social Security, 1975; and unpublished surveys). Average daily intakes of energy and most nutrients were not consistently less in children from large families or in those from Registrar General social classes IV and V. Intakes of vitamin C did show a consistent decrease with increasing family size and fall in Registrar General social class, but there were no signs of deficiency in any of the children. Measurements of attained height and weight showed the family size and social class trends to which reference has already been made.

In the 1967/68 survey of elderly people about 3 per cent of subjects over the age of 65 years were thought to be undernourished, and in most of these the poor nutritional status was associated with non-nutritional clinical disease (Department of Health and Social Security, 1972). Two of the participants had scurvy, and in two other subjects scurvy was suspected. This supports the fact that vitamin C deficiency although rare in this country can occur in elderly people, often in those who are widowed or living alone. The examining physicians agreed that there was a small problem of vitamin D deficiency, especially

Table 6. Department of Health and Social Security nutrition surveys

Year of survey	Subjects	Age (years)	No. in sample	Information collected					
				Socio-economic	Dietary 7 days weighed	Medical assess-ment	Anthropometry		
							Ht	Wt	Skinfold
1967-68	Preschoolchildren	½–4½	1321	+	+	about 10%	+	+	+
1971	Schoolchildren	10–11	321	+	+	+	+	+	+
1969-70	One parent families	14–15	178	+	+	+	+	+	+
1970-71	Schoolchildren	14–15	792	+	+	+	+	+	+
1967-68	Pregnant women		435	+	+	+	+	+	+
1967-68	Elderly*	65 and over	879	+	+	+	+	+	+
1972-73	Elderly*	70 and over	433	+	+	+	+	+	+
1973-74	Elderly*	65 and over	1506	+	+	+	+	+	+
1977-78	Elderly*	75 and over	154	+	+	+	+	+	+

*Studies of the elderly also included biochemistry, haematology and radiology of the metacarpals among the housebound elderly. In the five year follow-up study all these findings were confirmed (Department of Health and Social Security, 1979*b*)*. The number of subjects who were thought to be malnourished had increased to 7 per cent (26 of 365 subjects) as might be expected in a sample which was five years older. In all except one of the malnourished subjects undernutrition was associated with non-nutritional clinical disease. Social factors, such as bereavement, were also of importance.

Special studies

In the assessement of nutritional status, special studies have at times to be made either because the interpretation of survey information is incomplete until the significance of some findings has been elucidated, or because other workers report findings which indicate malnutrition. Assertions that intakes of dietary iron might be too small led to studies of anaemia in young children (MacWilliam, 1968) and in women (Elwood, 1968). Reports that schoolchildren and patients in geriatric hospitals were suffering from deficiencies of vitamin B and C led to feeding trials in which schoolchildren were randomly divided into a control and an experimental group which was given the vitamins by mouth (Yudkin *et al.*, 1970); and to a study in five London hospitals of the effects of vitamin supplements given in a double-blind trial to geriatric patients who were said to show the signs of deficiency (Berry & Darke, 1972). In none of these studies were the assertions confirmed.

In October 1970, the Government announced changes in the provision of welfare milk, school milk and school meals to be effective from April, 1971. The benefit of a daily pint of milk available at half price to all pregnant women and children under five years of age and free to the poor had been introduced with the Welfare Food Scheme in the 1940s. But from 1971 onwards the benefit was withdrawn from those who could afford to pay, and at the same time the number of expectant or lactating mothers, and of large families with preschool-children who received one pint of milk free of charge, was increased. Free school milk, one third of a pint daily on each day of the school year, had been withdrawn from the junior sections of primary schools. School milk was continued for all children up to the end of the school year in which they attained their seventh birthday, for all handicapped children and for all those of any age whom area medical officers said required milk for special medical reasons. The price of school meals was also increased.

The effects of these changes, if any, on nutritional status could not be readily foretold. They were likely to be small and depended on what food, if anything, replaced the cheap milk in the diet. Special studies were commissioned in 1971/72 to monitor the effects of the changes. The studies included growth of preschoolchildren and schoolchildren, the health of expectant mothers during pregnancy and growth and development of the infants born to them (Department of Health and Social Security, 1973). The studies were set up in the first place for a period of five years since any effect might take some time to become detectable. It was also recognised that long-term surveillance of growth was essential in order to provide evidence of nutritional status upon which future Government policy could be based. A report of these studies will be published.

**For further details see p. 126.*

In 1971/72 reports appeared in the medical press of an increase in the number of bottle-fed infants admitted to hospital with gastro-enteritis which proved to be associated with hypernatraemic dehydration. As a result a working party was set up to investigate infant feeding practice in the United Kingdom. This led to the publication of a report entitled *Present day practice in infant feeding* (Department of Health and Social Security, 1974) which set out clearly that breast feeding should be encouraged, and that unmodified cows' milk even when fortified with iron and vitamins was not a suitable feed for infants below the age of six months especially if prepared so that feeds were over-concentrated. As a result, from Feb. 1977 infant foods based on unmodified cows' milk, including National Dried Milk, were no longer allowed to be marketed and arrangements were made for the low-solute infant milks to be available free to those in receipt of welfare milk tokens for the first year of life. A special study of infant feeding practice was commissioned from the Office of Population Censuses and Surveys (Martin, 1978). This study has revealed attitudes and practice which must be changed by education if breast feeding is to be promoted and the best nutritional status assured for the young infant. The study was intended to be the first of a series made at intervals in order to monitor infant feeding practice. The 1974 report, referred to above, is now in many respects out-of-date and is being rewritten.

An assessment of nutritional status must include the diseases of overnutrition or of an imbalance of nutrients, that is to say, the diseases associated with what has come to be known as the 'Western type diet of an affluent society', affluent at least by comparison with two-thirds of the world. Until the economic recession of the past few years, obesity was thought to be the most common manifestation of malnutrition in the United Kingdom, but there is some evidence from local surveys that the number of overweight people is now less. A survey of adult height and weight is planned for 1980.

Conclusion

Although there is a problem of deficiency of vitamin D, and perhaps also of vitamin C, among minority groups of the population, and a quantitatively unknown problem of obesity, these problems are small compared with those of some countries. The nutritional status of the United Kingdom is in general 'good' and where it is not, lack of knowledge and mismanagement are the 'cause' of the deficiency rather than true poverty or lack of available food. Methods of assessing nutritional status are piece-meal and will continue to rely on food supply and health statistics, on in-depth nutrition surveys and on ad hoc studies unless and until some simpler assessment for large-scale use is found.

References

Arneil, G.C. (1975): *Proc. Nutr. Soc.* **34**, 101-109.

Berry, W.T.C. & Darke, S.J. (1972): *Age & Ageing* **1**, 177-181.

British Medical Association (1950): *Report of the Committee on Nutrition.* London: BMA.

Dawson, K.P. & Mondhe, M.S. (1972): *Practitioner* **208**, 789-791.

Department of Health and Social Security (1969): *Recommended intakes of nutrients for the United Kingdom.* Rep. Publ. Hlth Med. Subj. No. 120. London: HMSO.

Department of Health and Social Security (1972): *A nutrition survey of the elderly.* Rep. Hlth Soc. Subj. No. 3. London: HMSO.

Department of Health and Social Security (1973): *First report by the Sub-Committee on Nutritional Surveillance.* Rep. Hlth Soc. Subj. No. 6. London: HMSO.

Department of Health and Social Security (1974): *Present-day practice in infant feeding.* Rep. Hlth Soc. Subj. No. 9. London: HMSO.

Department of Health and Social Security (1975): *A nutrition survey of preschoolchildren.* Rep. Hlth Soc. Subj. No. 10. London: HMSO.

Department of Health and Social Security (1979*a*): *Recommended daily amounts of food energy and nutrients for groups of people in the United Kingdom.* Rep. Hlth Soc. Subj. No. 15. London: HMSO.

Department of Health and Social Security (1979*b*): *Nutrition and health in old age.* Rep. Hlth Soc. Subj. No. 16. London: HMSO.

Department of Health and Social Security (1980): *Rickets and osteomalacia.* London: HMSO (In press).

Elwood, P.C. (1968): *Proc. Nutr. Soc.* 27, 14-23.

MacWilliam, K. (1968): *Haemoglobin levels in young children.* Rep. Publ. Hlth Med. Subj. No. 118. Appendix H. London: HMSO.

Martin, J. (1978): *Infant feeding 1975 : attitudes and practice in England and Wales.* Office of Population Censuses and Surveys : Social Survey Division. London: HMSO.

Ministry of Agriculture, Fisheries and Food (1960): *Domestic food consumption and expenditure : 1958,* Annual Report of the National Food Survey Committee. London: HMSO.

Ministry of Agriculture, Fisheries and Food (1970): *Household food consumption and expenditure : 1968.* Annual Report of the National Food Survey Committee. London: HMSO.

Ministry of Agriculture, Fisheries and Food (1979): *British Business* 37, 573.

Ministry of Agriculture, Fisheries and Food (1980): *Household food consumption and expenditure : 1978.* Annual Report of the National Food Survey Committee; London: HMSO.

Ministry of Health (1968): *A pilot survey of the nutrition of young children in 1963.* Rep. Publ. Hlth Med. Subj. No. 118. London: HMSO.

Office of Population Censuses and Surveys : Social Surveys Division (1977): *The general household survey, 1974.* London: HMSO.

Office of Population and Surveys (1975, 1978, 1979): *Population trends. Nos 1, 12, 18. Vital statistics.* London: HMSO

Sosa, R., Kennell, J.H., Klaus, M. & Urrutia, J.J. (1976): In *Breast feeding and the mother,* p. 179. Ciba Foundation Symposium 45. Amsterdam: Elsevier.

Weiner, J.S. & Lourie, J.A. (1969): *Human biology. A guide to field methods.* IBP Handbook, No. 9. Oxford and Edinburgh: Blackwell Scientific.

Yudkin, J., Norman, D.H., Wilkinson, M.E. & Berry, W.T.C. (1970): *Proc. Nutr. Soc.* 29, 8A.

11

Recommended dietary intakes

Erica F. Wheeler.

Introduction

Advice and recommendations about diet have been exchanged from very early on in our history. The ancient Egyptians believed that many disorders arose in the alimentary tract and recommended the use of figs and other fruits to maintain a regular bowel habit. The writer of *Proverbs* noted that 'Better is a dry morsel with quiet, than a house full of feasting with strife'. The famous medical faculty which flourished in Salerno in the Middle Ages commended a cereal (bread) and milk as a food mixture particularly suitable for babies (Tannahill, 1975). Today, almost identical advice is still being given by doctors and nutritionists, for the good reason that it is still valid and useful.

However, the recommendations mainly considered in this chapter are more precise than these general empirical precepts on food and diet which the human race has developed over many centuries. Ever since the first scientific studies of the relationship between specific nutrients and physical health, nutrition scientists have attempted to answer the question: 'How much of any nutrient need a healthy person have?' Before recommended intakes are considered in detail, it is useful to ask some general questions about them. This chapter does not give a complete list of any set of recommended intakes, and should be read in conjunction with the tables published by The Food and Agriculture Organisation (FAO) and the (UK) Department of Health and Social Security (DHSS) – see references.

Why are tables of recommended intakes prepared?

They are most commonly intended to be used for assessing the results of dietary surveys, although, as will be shown below, this raises various statistical problems. When a survey shows that a certain group of people consume a certain amount of, say, protein, recommended intake figures are invoked as a yardstick by which the intakes are judged. Large scale surveys commissioned by government (such as the UK National Food Survey) are often intended to show whether certain sections of the population are receiving adequate diets, as well as to monitor trends in food consumption and choice. Government policy on food subsidies, imports and distribution may be partly influenced by what is known about the adequacy of diets. Another reason given for preparing these tables is that they may be used in calculating ration scales and menus for institutions such as hospitals, schools, prisons and barracks. (In the writer's experience, however, ration scales are usually drawn up on the basis of experience and food availability.) Probably the principal use made of 'recommended intakes' is to assess dietary survey findings, both for individuals and for groups.

Who prepares them?
Usually a committee of interested scientists convened either by the agriculture or health ministry of a country, or by an international agency such as the Food and Agriculture Organisation (FAO). The examples of recommended intakes quoted in this chapter are drawn from FAO reports unless otherwise stated (FAO 1961, 1967, 1970 and 1973). The advantage of using international standard figures is that the results of surveys from different countries can then be compared on the same basis.

Are they necessary?
It is impossible to answer this question before making the distinction between *requirements* and *recommendations,* as follows.

Minimum physiological requirements
Every human being needs certain essential nutrients; and for each there is a minimum amount which must be absorbed daily by the body in order to maintain health. This minimum amount can never by exactly and precisely defined even for one individual, since each of us varies from day to day in activity and rate of metabolism. But for groups of similar persons (eg adult non-pregnant non-lactating women) it is reasonable to define a theoretical minimum intake, such that someone having less of the nutrient would almost certainly develop signs of deficiency.

In order to estimate the minimum requirement for a nutrient, something must be known about its function and metabolism. Figure 1 shows schematically the pathways of a nutrient through the body, and indicates the information which is needed in order to estimate requirements. In its simplest form this can be expressed as:

$$\text{Minimum requirements} = \text{urinary loss} + \text{faecal loss} + \text{other losses} + \text{needs for growth, foetus and lactation where appropriate}$$

$$\text{or } R = U + F + O + (G) + (L)$$

but there are two main problem areas. Faecal and urinary losses vary according to intake, so how are they to be estimated? and faecal losses especially may be affected by other food constituents, such as phytic acid, which alters the digestibility of minerals. Secondly, some nutrients (eg thiamin) are metabolised and excreted in another form, so it is not sufficient only to measure thiamin excretion. A number of different techniques have been used for estimating the

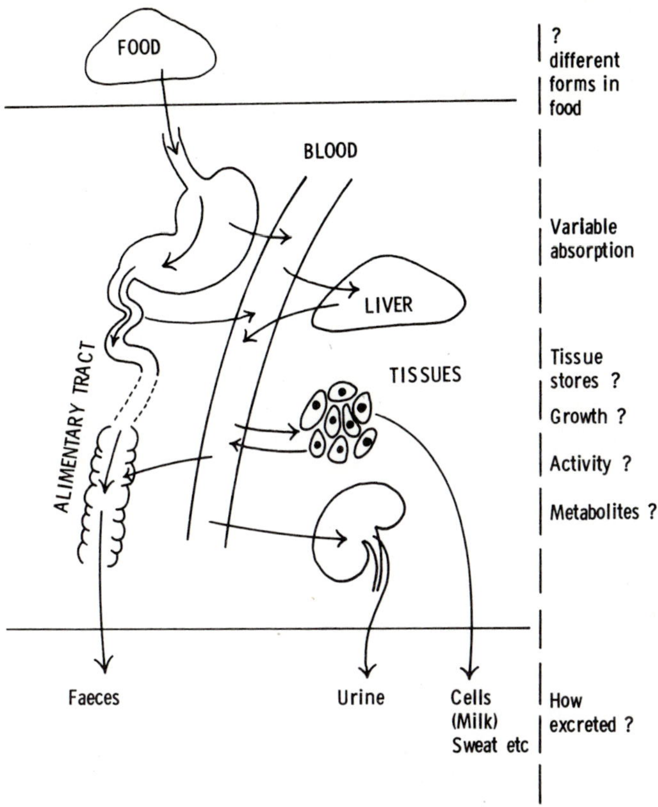

Fig. 1. Information needed about body use and losses of nutrients

requirement for different nutrients, and Table 1 summarises these. Essentially the aim is, if possible, to estimate losses of the nutrient from the body, and to discover the amount of nutrient necessary to maintain equilibrium. In adults, 'equilibrium' implies zero weight gain; in children, an acceptable rate of growth such as that described by the 'Harvard' growth standards (Nelson, Vaughan & McKay, 1969).

The clearest example of this approach is a UK committee's estimate of adult nitrogen (protein) requirements (DHSS, 1969). The requirement figures for different types of people were built up by the 'factorial method' of collecting separate estimates of U, F, O, G, and L and combining them. The problem of variable urinary and faecal losses was met by using data for *'obligatory losses'*, ie the amount excreted in urine, sweat and faeces by individuals on nitrogen-free diets. The obligatory loss reflects the inevitable shedding of cells, and production of enzymes and other secretions, and the nitrogen released as urea when body proteins are metabolised. Numerous measurements have been made of obligatory nitrogen losses in adults, and the committee was able to make a synthesis of these. An arbitrary factor of 10 per cent was added to make allowance for normal variation between individuals (see below), thus the adult N requirement was computed as: $R = (U + F + O) \times 1.1$.

Practical difficulties arise in applying this method to children and to pregnant

Table 1. Methods which have been used to estimate minimum physiological requirements for nutrients

Method	Nutrients
Metabolic studies	
Balance studies (intake needed to maintain equilibrium)	Nitrogen, calcium, iron
Measurement of obligatory losses	Nitrogen, iron
Controlled depletion-repletion experiments	Vitamin A, thiamin, vitamin A riboflavin, niacin, ascorbic acid
Urinary excretion and blood levels of metabolites	Thiamin
Use of radioactive isotopes to measure whole body turnover	Iron, vitamin B_{12}, ascorbic acid
Dietary and clinical studies	
Amount of nutrient needed to reverse clinical signs of deficiency	Thiamin, vitamin B_{12}, folic acid, vitamin D
Comparison of habitual intakes in clinically deficiency and healthy populations	Vitamin A, thiamin, riboflavin, niacin, ascorbic acid, vitamin D
Children	
Estimates of amount laid down during growth	Nitrogen, calcium
Estimates of amounts supplied in breast milk	All nutrients

and lactating women: obviously they cannot be given nitrogen-free diets. Some measurements have been made in children receiving low-protein diets for a short time, but most of the requirement figures are based on analysis of the nitrogen content of milk, of the foetus and of growing tissue, added on to estimated obligatory losses. Clearly, the precision attained by nitrogen-free diet experiments in adults can never be gained with children.

The values for requirements obtained by the factorial method can be checked by the results of *balance studies*. Here an individual is given a daily food intake which contains a known amount of nutrient; all excreta are collected and analysed, and over a period the sum Balance = intake − (F + U + O) is calculated. An intake close to the minimum requirement should result in zero balance, or an equilibrium state, in adults. In children, there should be a positive value for the balance, corresponding to the normal growth rate for that age. This method has been used to establish infants' requirements for minerals and nitrogen. It has also been used to estimate adult minimum requirements for calcium.

The measurement of excretory losses on a diet free of the nutrient being considered is sometimes described as 'depletion', since the procedure may considerably deplete the body stores of certain nutrients. For a number of the vitamins, where faecal and skin excretion is practically nil, obligatory urinary excretion has been measured in depletion experiments and used as an estimate of the minimum requirement. The time needed to deplete body stores varies, but the vitamin-free diet must be continued until urinary excretion stops falling and reaches a steady 'plateau' level, when body stores are being drawn upon to supply the minimum necessary amount of vitamin. This method has been used for several of the 'B' group of vitamins (see Table 1). However, for some other vitamins urinary excretion is not a good measure of obligatory loss: ascorbic acid disappears from the urine altogether in depletion, and vitamins D and A are not excreted at all by this route. For vitamin A and ascorbic acid, plasma levels falling to a plateau were taken to indicate that a minimal amount of vitamin was being used up: and the least dose necessary to bring about an increase, was taken as the minimum requirement: this is a *depletion-repletion* technique. This has been done in a controlled manner with adult volunteers by depleting them until they become clinically deficient, and then finding the least amount of nutrient necessary to reverse their symptoms. Well-known experiments along these lines were conducted with non-combatant volunteers during World War II, in respect of vitamins A and C (Medical Research Council, 1949, 1953).

To take one nutrient as an example, thiamin requirements have been mainly established by depletion-repletion experiments and confirmed by population diet studies. The value found in tables thus represents a synthesis of the results of many measurements, of different types. Thiamin requirements are usually expressed 'per 1000 kilocalories' or 'per 1000 kiloJoules'. This is a useful convention, sometimes referred to as '*nutrient density*', which enables the requirements of some nutrients (mainly those concerned in energy metabolism) to be expressed concisely and generally.

There are a number of nutrients (such as, sodium, magnesium, vitamin B_6, vitamin E, to give some examples) for which the requirements have not been studied in such detail as those previously mentioned because dietary deficiencies rarely occur. In practice nobody worries about the sodium or vitamin K level in the UK adult diet. A dietitian may need to maintain a patient on a 'minimal potassium' diet, or something similar; but in such a case the patient's clinical and biochemical state would be carefully monitored and used as a guide, rather than a minimum requirement figure.

Statistical problems, and 'safe levels'

Estimates of minimal physiological requirements are, as we have seen, based on numerous measurements, and the final figure may be seen as a mean value for a group, such as 1 to 3-year-old children or adult men. What is the standard deviation around this mean? As Figure 2 indicates, it is usually assumed to be 10-15 per cent because this is the observed standard deviation of adult 'basal' metabolic rates (Shock *et al.*, 1963). Thus, the addition of 10-30 per cent which is commonly made to requirement figures 'to allow for variation' represents + 1 or + 2 standard deviations. The mean value plus 2 s.d. is often referred to as a '*safe level of intake*' since, from classical statistical theory, this amount is supposed to cover the needs of 97 per cent of the population. This term may not be the ideal one, but it is in use.

Suppose the distribution of requirements indicated in Fig. 2 represents the thiamin requirements of 1 to 3-year-old children. If we find in a survey that child

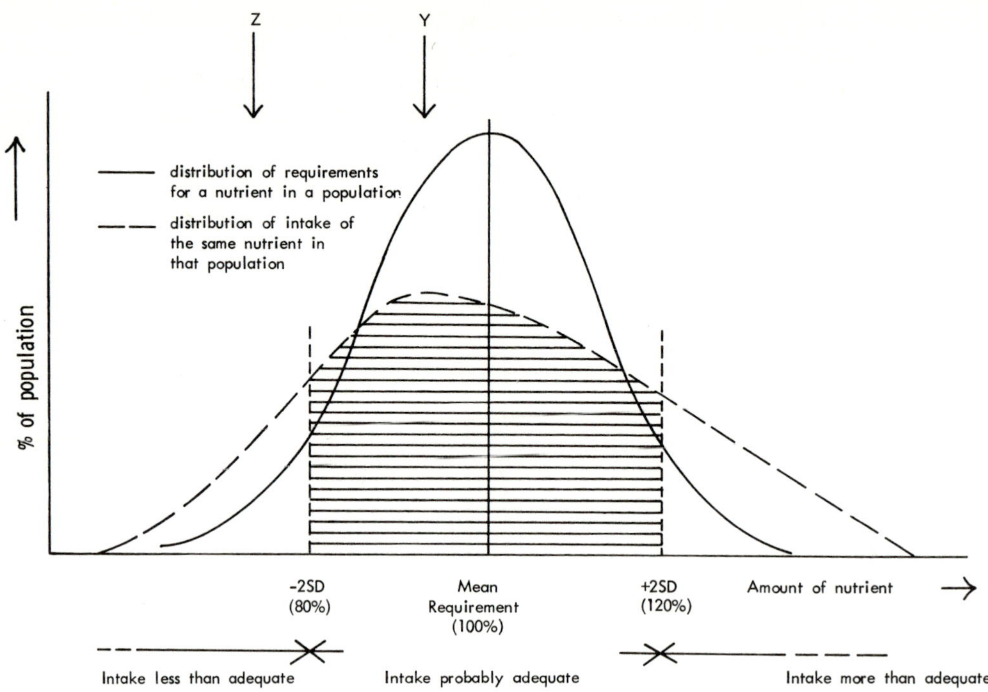

Fig. 2. Distribution of the intakes and requirements of a nutrient in a hypothetical population

Y has an intake of 90 per cent of the group requirement, while for child Z the intake is 75 per cent, what can we conclude? We do not know the exact requirements of either child; we only know that there is a high probability that both Y and Z require something between 80 per cent and 120 per cent of the mean requirement. So for child Y, we do not actually know whether his intake is adequate or not. An intake equal to (or 100 per cent of) the requirement means a 50 per cent probability (5 chances in 10), that the intake is adequate. At 90 per cent, the probability is 16 per cent, or nearly 2 chances in 10, that the intake is equal to or greater than his requirements. On the other hand, child Z's intake is well below the 80 per cent - 120 per cent 'range of possible adequacy' and, if his intake is habitually so low, he will almost certainly show clinical signs of deficiency.

If instead of individual children's intakes we have the mean intake of a group, we can only make positive statements that the intakes are adequate if they all lie above 120 per cent of mean requirements. If not, there is certainly a chance that some individuals have intakes less than requirement; but they cannot be identified unless the group data are disaggregated and they are considered individually. In presenting the results of a survey it is more meaningful to count up and identify individuals whose intakes fall below a certain level, than to lump them all together in a group mean intake.

Recommended intakes

Having discussed physiological minimum requirements, which are measured and reasonably well understood quantities, we now arrive at 'recommended intakes'. These also represent the deliberations of the expert committees mentioned in the introduction, but they are now responding not to the question 'What is the least amount of nutrient which people need to consume?' but 'how much *should* they consume?' The recommended intake is often constructed because there is felt to be a need to advise or instruct people about a 'good', 'average' or 'optimal' diet, rather than informing them about the least amount which will preserve their health.

This introduces a new dimension into the picture. If we are no longer simply considering what people need, but what we think they would like to have, or should have, there is much more scope for differences of opinion, and much more difficulty in reconciling the views of different authorities. Also, clearly, there is no particular scientific basis for the recommendations, *unless* they are defined as the 'safe level', ie the minimum requirement plus 2 standard deviations. Otherwise, they may simply represent common practice or opinion. A number of possible ways of constructing recommended allowances, (see Table 2) are:

Table 2. The relationship between Minimum Requirements (MR), and Recommended Allowances (RA) for some nutrients, as laid down by various authorities. (References: FAO 1967, 1970 and 1973; DHSS 1969; NAS-NRC, 1968).

Nutrient and source	Relationship
PROTEIN (Nitrogen)	
International (FAO)	RA = MR + 30%
UK	RA = 10% of total energy, as in typical diets
ASCORBIC ACID	
International (FAO), UK	RA = MR x 3
USA	RA = MR x 7
IRON	
International (FAO)	RA = MR x 5 – MR x 10, depending on type of diet and absorption
UK	RA = MR x 10
VITAMIN D	
International (FAO), UK	MR unknown. RA derived from studies of typical diets
THIAMIN, RIBOFLAVIN AND NIACIN	
International (FAO)	RA = MR + 20% (ie, safe level)

1. To take the 'safe level' as the recommended intake. FAO has done this for thiamin, riboflavin and niacin.
2. To adopt the 'safe level' approach but to add a further margin, allowing for poor absorption (iron, calcium) or, in the case or protein, for differences in the protein quality of diets.
3. To relate the recommendation to the minimum requirement, but to allow a

very large margin for individual variation, far more than ± 20 per cent. This has been done by FAO for ascorbic acid and folic acid. There is no obvious reason for selecting these margins of error.

4. To recommend the amounts used in daily average diets. FAO has done this for vitamin D, for which the minimum requirement is not known. A UK committee (DHSS, 1969) recommended a protein intake which enshrines the structure of the typical British diet at that time: ie with 10 per cent of dietary energy derived from protein. This gives rise to values roughly double the minimum requirement; presumably if the British altered their dietary habits and consumed more protein, the recommendation would be brought into line. At present, recommended intakes for protein in Europe vary from 37 g/day in Spain to 105 in Roumania (Zollner, Wolfran & Keller, 1977). There is no such differential in minimum requirements between the peoples of these two countries. Protein recommended intakes in particular have been used to express desirable standards of living rather than physiological need.

5. To advocate a level of intake which is supposed to maintain body stores of the vitamin at a particular high level. The amount of ascorbic acid in plasma for example, can vary between 0.2 and 2.0 mg/100 ml. The US recommended intake is designed to maintain a high level in plasma and cells (NAS-NRC, 1968). Other authorities, which are unconvinced of the benefits of saturating cells with ascorbic acid, have recommended lower intakes.

The variation in methods of constructing recommended intake tables, and the discrepancies between them and minimal physiological requirements, are therefore considerable and should be borne in mind when they are consulted.

Unless the approaches become more standardised, the recommendations are likely to remain diverse. A lot of confusion has already arisen over terminology. Some tables (such as those published by FAO) are entitled 'Requirements of ....', when in fact the contents are recommended intakes, and students and other users tend to make use of the two terms as if they were interchangeable. One hears diets being pronounced 'inadequate' or 'deficient' because their nutrient value falls below some *recommended value* which is considerably higher than the *minimum.*

Energy: the special case

The requirements for most nutrients are related to body weight, thus, if one loses a lot of weight, technically one's individual vitamin and protein requirements fall. Also, increased activity implies an increased requirement for nutrients concerned in metabolism. These variations can be contained within the range of values for a particular age/sex group. However, for energy (and therefore for the main energy-yielding nutrients, fat and carbohydrate) there is such an interaction between body stores, physical activity, intake and expenditure that a minimum requirement for energy is almost impossible to define. The 'basal metabolic rate' (BMR) is the nearest to a standardised measure of requirement; and it has been suggested that a minimum level of intake should be at least 1.5 times this, to allow for the energy expenditure involved in meal-eating and minimal physical activity. All that can be said about energy intakes is that if a group of people had an energy intake less than 1.5 times the BMR appropriate to their sex and average weight, most of them must be either totally inactive, or losing weight.

'Recommended intakes' for energy are derived from measurements of the diets consumed by healthy people at varying weights and activity levels. Obviously an individual having an intake below the recommended intake is not necessarily deficient since the recommendation is a group average. In fact the best way of finding out whether someone is in energy deficit is to weigh them. Energy 'recommendations' simply represent typical diets, and should be used as such.

Are recommended intakes necessary?

We can now return to the earlier question 'Are they necessary?' and apply it to both minimum requirements, and recommended intakes. For *minimum requirements* and their associated safe levels, there is certainly a useful role. In the evaluation of nutrition problems at any level, individual, local or national, it is often necessary to ask 'Does the diet supply sufficient nutrients?', as a supplementary to questions about the clinical and biochemical status of individuals. For this, some requirement figure is needed as a cut-off point. More work is needed on some nutrients, especially vitamin D, folic acid and calcium, in order to specify the requirement better. But for many nutrients, the data are there.

As well as the better definition of some requirement figures, there is also a need for some systematic work connecting the degree to which a dietary intake falls below the requirement with the risks incurred by the consumer of the diet. At present we can only guess at the risk to an individual of consuming, say, a low iron diet, in terms of the chances of becoming severely anaemic. What kind of risk do I take by refusing to eat 'red meat, legumes and dark green leafy vegetables'? Nobody knows.

Are *recommended intakes* or allowances also necessary? The areas in which they are generally held to be useful are: the planning of menus and diets, the evaluation of surveys, and the development of Government policy on food supplies. For the first two of these, 'safe levels' based on minimum requirement would not only be perfectly adequate, but would reduce some of the confusion attached to interpretation. If data are available on, for instance the ascorbic acid intakes of old age pensioners in the North-East of England, we need to know how many receive intakes below the 'safe level': in other words, how many are in the area of potential deficiency? To define a higher 'recommended intake' only invites the question 'so what?' if we find that most old people, for instance, are not receiving it – because we do not know the significance of the finding. If what we really want is an index of the *quality* of diet, or the *standard of living* of the elderly, then an appropriate index might be constructed. But this should not be a nutritional index, and should not be described as such. It would be a way of using dietary data to describe one aspect of a socio-economic concept, ie standard of living. A relatively low-protein or low-ascorbic acid intake, although nutritionally adequate, may indeed be a 'poor man's diet', and unacceptable for that reason. However, we should not invoke a non-existent nutritional deficiency when what we are really confronting is social deprivation. In order to prevent this confusion it would be better to use physiological estimates of requirement as nutritional yardsticks, and devise specific indices for assessing the quality and social value of diets. Such an index might be based on what the community feels is 'good' or socially acceptable. In the UK, it might include the number of meals eaten daily, the number of certain key indicator foods consumed, and the proportion of disposable income spent on food, for example.

A word of warning must be inserted at this point. Although there is a need for a non-nutritional way of assessing a meal pattern, this should not be seen simply as a method (such as the 'Four Food Group Plan' in the USA) of approximating to an assessment of nutrient intake. It should provide a judgement of the social value of the diet independently of its nutritional value; of the extent to which the diet satisfies the consumers' aspirations and makes them feel that their standard of living is a reasonable one.

A further problem involved in the use of recommended intake figures is expressed by suggestion that upper levels, as well as lower levels, of intake should be set, and that for some foods and nutrients (especially saturated fat and sugar) government policy on imports and prices should reflect a discouraging attitude to high intakes. This suggestion is exemplified in the 'Dietary Goals' agreed by the US Senate in 1977 (US Senate Committee on Nutrition and Human Needs, 1977). Here again we have two problems: that we cannot actually quantify the risk associated with consuming a certain level of fat or sugar, and that public opinion on 'What is an acceptable and desirable diet' flatly contradicts the recommendation. Here again nutritional knowledge, nutritional opinions, and various social values have become tangled together. At present we have not sufficient knowledge to prescribe 'ceilings' on intakes of most nutrients. In any case, this may not prove to be acceptable in our society; advice to an individual on his obesity is one thing, but prescription of the dietary pattern of a whole nation of obese and non-obese people is another.

In summary, it appears that recommended intakes or allowances have no function which could not be fulfilled somewhat better by physiological requirement figures: and that the acceptance of two, three or more prescribed levels of nutrient intake has led to a good deal of double-talk when intakes are being compared with 'standards'. Assessments of the 'goodness' or social acceptability of diets should be made using non-nutritional criteria. Both the more accurate definition of certain minimum requirements, and the compilation of social indices of diet quality, are areas of study worth exploring further.

References

DHSS (1969): *Recommended intakes of nutrients for the United Kingdom.* Rep. Publ. Hlth Med. Subj. No. 120. London: HMSO.

FAO (1961): *Calcium requirements.* FAO Nutr. Mtgs Rep. Ser. No. 30. Rome: FAO.

FAO (1967): *Requirements of vitamin A, thiamine, riboflavin and niacin.* FAO Nutr. Mtgs Rep. Ser. No. 41. Rome: FAO.

FAO (1970): *Requirements of ascorbic acid, vitamin D, vitamin B_{12}, folate and iron.* FAO Nutr. Mtgs Rep. Ser. No. 47. Rome: FAO.

FAO (1973): *Energy and protein requirements.* FAO Nutr. Mtgs Rep. Ser. No. 52. Rome: FAO.

Medical Research Council (1949): *Spec. Rep. Ser. No. 264.* London: HMSO.

Medical Research Council (1953): *Spec. Rep. Ser. No. 280.* London: HMSO.
NAS-NRC (1968): *Recommended dietary allowances.* Washington DC: NAS.
Nelson, W.E., Vaughan, V.C. & McKay, R.J. (1969): *Textbook of pediatrics.* London: Saunders.
Shock, N.W., Watkin, D.M., Yiengst, M.J., Norris, A.H., Gaffney, G.W., Gregarman, R.I. & Falzone, J.A. (1963): *J. Gerontol.* 18, 1.
Tannahill, R. (1975): *Food in history.* London: Methuen.
US Senate Committee on Nutrition and Human Needs (1977): *Dietary Goals for the United States.* Washington DC: Govt. Ptg Office.
Zollner, N., Wolfram, G. & Keller, C. Editors (1977): *Second European Nutrition Conference:* main papers. Karger, Basel.

Bibliographic note

The most recent tables of *recommended intakes* for the UK are 'Recommended daily amounts of food energy and nutrients for groups of people in the United Kingdom' (DHSS Report on Health and Social Subjects: 15, 1979). Strictly speaking the only data on *minimum requirements* applicable to the UK are the FAO publications discussed in the text.
A revised (ninth) edition of 'Recommended dietary allowances' is in the press (1980) from Food and Nutrition Board, National Academy of Sciences - National Research Council, Washington DC. (See J. Am. Diet. Ass. 1979, 75, 623-625 for advance details of the tables).

The authors

Margaret ASHWELL, PhD: Division of Clinical Sciences, Clinical Research Centre, Watford Road, Harrow HA1 3UJ, Middlesex.

Sheila T. CALLENDER, MD, DSc, FRCP: Nuffield Department of Clinical Medicine, John Radcliffe Hospital, Headington, Oxford OX3 9DU.

I. CHANARIN, MD, FRCPath: Department of Haematology, Northwick Park Hospital and Clinical Research Centre, Watford Road, Harrow HA1 3UJ, Middlesex.

Merril DURRANT, BSc: Division of Clinical Sciences, Clinical Research Centre, Watford Road, Harrow HA1 3UJ, Middlesex.

Sylvia J. DARKE, MSc, MBChB: Department of Health and Social Security, Alexander Fleming House, London SE1 6BY.

M. A. EASTWOOD, MSc, FRCP Edin.: Wolfson Laboratories, Gastrointestinal Unit, Western General Hospital, Edinburgh EH4 2XU.

A. N. EXTON-SMITH, MD, FRCP: Barlow Professor of Geriatric Medicine, University College Hospital Medical School, London, at St. Pancras Hospital.

J. S. GARROW, PhD, MD, FRCP Edin: Division of Clinical Sciences, Clinical Research Centre, Watford Road, Harrow HA1 3UJ, Middlesex.

A. N. HOWARD, PhD: Department of Medicine, University of Cambridge, Addenbrroke's Hospital, Hills Road, Cambridge CB2 2QQ.

R. HUGHES, PhD, FIBiol: Department of Applied Biology, University of Wales, University Institute of Science and Technology, Cardiff, Wales.

Ian MACDONALD, MD, DSc, FIBiol: Professor of Applied Physiology, Department of Physiology, Guy's Hospital Medical School, London SE1 9RT.

B. E. C. NORDIN, DSc, PhD, MD, FRCP: Director, MRC Mineral Metabolism Unit, and Professor of Mineral Metabolism, Martin Wing, General Infirmary, St. George Street, Leeds LS1 3RX.

Penelope WARWICK, PhD: Division of Clinical Sciences, Clinical Research Centre, Watford Road, Harrow HA1 3UJ, Middlesex.

Erica F. WHEELER, BSc, MPhil: Department of Human Nutrition, London School of Hygiene and Tropical Medicine, Keppel Street, London WC1E 7HT.

Index